A GUIDE TO
SPORTS AND INJURY
MANAGEMENT

Commissioning Editors: Claire Wilson, Rita Demetriou-Swanwick
Development Editor: Sally Davies
Project Manager: Joannah Duncan
Designer/Design Direction: Charles Gray
Illustration Manager: Merlyn Harvey
Illustrator: Chartwell, Cactus

A GUIDE TO
SPORTS AND INJURY
MANAGEMENT

Mike Bundy MBBS MRCGP DipSportsMed(Bath) FFSEM(UK)
Sports Physician, Pure Sports Medicine, Kensington, London, UK

Andy Leaver BSc(Hons) MCSP SRP
Head Physiotherapist, Bath Rugby Club, Bath, UK

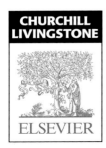

Edinburgh London New York Oxford Philadelphia St Louis Sydney Toronto 2010

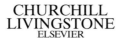

CHURCHILL
LIVINGSTONE
ELSEVIER

ISBN 978 0 443 06813 3

British Library Cataloguing in Publication Data
A catalogue record for this book is available from the British Library

Library of Congress Cataloging in Publication Data
A catalog record for this book is available from the Library of Congress

Printed in China

617.1027
B942

Contents

The DVD accompanying this text includes video sequences of all the techniques and exercises indicated in the text by the icon. To look at the video for a given technique, click on the relevant icon in the contents list on the DVD. The DVD is designed to be used in conjunction with the text and not as a stand-alone product.

DVD CONTENTS

The DVD accompanying this text contains:

The Interactive Diagnosis Tool
Video clips
Multiple Choice Questions relating to
    each chapter in the book

The Interactive Diagnosis Tool

The tool aids diagnosis of common
    injuries and opens as a colour image
    of the selected part of the human
    body (e.g. ankle and foot). The user
    clicks onto the image to bring on
    screen a more detailed anatomical
    drawing of that body area. The user
    can choose to view the ankle from
    anterior, inferior, lateral, medial and
    posterior views.
Within each of these views the user
    moves the cursor over the image and
    as trigger points on the image are
    highlighted the various diagnoses pop
    up on screen. The diagnoses are split
    into acute (red), chronic (blue) and
    referred (green) diagnoses. There are
    over 200 common injuries diagnoses
    included in the tool.

COMMON INJURIES

Ankle and foot
Anterior view
Forefoot (anterior view)
Inferior view (sole of foot)
Lateral view
Medial view
Midfoot (anterior view)
Posterior view

Buttock
Posterior view (lumbar spine to mid
thigh)

Groin and pelvis
Anterior view
Lateral view
Posterior view

Knee
Anterior view
Lateral view
Medial view

Posterior view
Inferior view
Superior view
Acute

Lower leg
Anterior view
Posterior view

Shoulder
Anterior view
Posterior view

Spine
Cervical – posterior view
Lumbar and sacral – anterior/lateral/
    posterior views
Lumbar and sacral – posterior view
Thoracic – posterior view

Thigh
Anterior view
Posterior view

Upper limb
Anterior view
Medial view
Lateral view
Posterior view

Wrist and hand
Anterior view
Posterior view

VIDEO CLIPS
There are video sequences of all the
    techniques and exercises indicated in
    the text by the icon. To look at the
    video for a given technique, click on
    the relevant item in the contents list
    on the DVD.

Assessment of the ankle joint
Ankle dorsiflexion
Ankle eversion
Ankle inversion
Ankle plantar flexion
Anterior drawer test for the anterior
    talo-fibular ligament
Posterior impingement test
Syndesmosis test

Assessment of the knee joint
Anterior drawer test for the anterior
   cruciate ligament (ACL)
Dial test for the posterolateral corner
Lachman's test for the ACL
McMurray's test for the meniscii
Patello-femoral joint glides
Posterior drawer test for posterior
   cruciate ligament (PCL)
Posterior sag test for the PCL
Valgus stress test for the medial
   collateral knee ligament (MCL)
Varus stress test for the lateral collateral
   knee ligament (LCL)

Assessment of the hip joint
Hip flexion
Hip medial and lateral rotation
Ober's test
Quadrant test
Test for impingement of the anterior
   capsule of the hip
Thomas test

Lumbar spine assessment and lower limb nerve provocation tests
Lumbar flexion and extension
Slump test
Straight leg raise

Assessment of the sacroiliac joint (SIJ)
SIJ kinetic test – forward flexion
Stork test

Assessment of the elbow joint
Valgus stress test for the medial
   collateral elbow ligament (MCL)
Varus stress test for the lateral collateral
   elbow ligament (LCL)

Assessment of the shoulder joint
Apprehension and relocation tests
Empty and full can tests
Hawkins Kennedy test

Neers test
O'Briens test
Resisted empty and full can tests
Scapulohumeral rhythm
Sulcus test
The 'Scarf' acromioclavicular joint test

Upper limb nerve provocation tests
Upper limb tension test (ULTT 1) –
   median nerve bias
Upper limb tension test (ULTT 2) – radial
   nerve bias
Upper limb tension test (ULTT 3) – ulnar
   nerve bias

Assessment of lower limb stability and muscular control
One-legged squat

Warm-up stretching programmes
Dynamic stretching warm-up
Static stretch warm-up

Proprioception/balance exercises
BOSU hops
Single-leg BOSU balance
Single-leg BOSU squats

Weight training examples
Bench press
Squat

Rehabilitation exercises
Eccentric Achilles tendon exercises
Eccentric patella tendon exercises
Knee drives
Nordic hamstring exercises

Core stability exercises
Floor core exercises
Gym ball core exercises

Other
30-second neurological examination
Application of a cervical collar

Preface

As a training sports physician I felt there was a lack of teaching material that was both practical and which suited my way of visual learning. I was desperate to find a book or DVD that took me through symptoms, signs, investigation and management combined with a list of possible differential diagnoses that was visual and reflected how we manage patients in the clinic. I was pleased to find that after working together with Andy at London Irish Rugby Club he had a similar train of thought. We therefore hatched the idea of developing a book and DVD that was very practical, visual, and, most importantly, gave information from both a physician's and physiotherapist's perspective. The project has taken several years to develop and the final product will hopefully be of value to sports physicians, physiotherapists, osteopaths, chiropractors, sports masseurs and all those training in these fields as well as keen athletes.

Mike Bundy
London, 2009

Having worked as a physiotherapist in sport for a number of years, it has become very apparent that there are a vast number of clinical signs, tests, techniques and exercises that clinicians have to remember. While there are a number of other textbooks available, I have yet to find one that has taken me through the assessment techniques to the clinical findings and then to the rehabilitation techniques to treat the injury in an easy-to-follow and visual manner. Having worked with Mike for a number of years, we felt that we could produce a book which would provide clinicians with all the necessary information to accurately assess, diagnose and rehabilitate a wide variety of commonly occurring sports injuries in a new and exciting format. In doing so, we have incorporated photographs into the book and videoclips onto the interactive DVD to highlight a number of the important tests and exercises. We hope that all the clinicians who read this will find it very useful.

Andy Leaver
London, 2009

Acknowledgements

We would very much like to thank Chris West and Hannah Bundy for agreeing to be in the photographs and would also like to thank Sarah Mitchell, Sarah Bundy and Phil Leaver for all their help in taking the photographs and video clips.

M.B.
A.L.

Chapter | 1 |

Training and conditioning

© 2009 Elsevier Ltd, Inc, BV
DOI: 10.1016/B978-0-443-06813-3.00004-1

The conditioning of athletes is an area which has become very popular and that has made significant advances in recent years. It is an ever-changing discipline because there has been a much greater emphasis placed on athletes being at the peak of physical condition for their sporting event, whether this be by having a greater cardiovascular capacity or being 'fitter' or by being stronger. This has led to strength and conditioning coaches being widely employed in most sporting disciplines to devise training programmes to ensure that the athletes are at the peak of their physical condition so that they are able to compete at the best of their ability in their competitions or matches.

It is, however, an ever-changing area with new and different concepts being devised all the time in an attempt to push the boundaries of physical performance and give the athlete an edge over their competitors. This is achieved by the strength and conditioning staff analysing the specific demands of each individual competitor. The physical demands obviously differ between sports but they can also differ between team mates who play in different positions on the same team. For example, the strength and conditioning programme for a prop in rugby will be quite different to that of a winger on the same team because of the different physical demands placed on each of them in the game. Therefore, it is very important to remember that the programmes need to be tailored to the individual and should be sport-specific for the greatest benefits to occur. For example, a cyclist needs to cycle and sports which are running-based, such as football and rugby, need their athletes to run and so on.

This chapter will discuss some of the different training techniques that are being employed and give some examples of useful sessions for some athletes.

AEROBIC TRAINING

Aerobic training is simply where oxygen is present and is used to generate energy when the glycogen stores in the muscles are broken down to produce glucose and hence allow muscle contractions to continue. It is the most common type of training and that done by members of the public who are trying to 'keep fit'. This is because it has been shown to have numerous health benefits:

- It improves the efficiency and strength of the cardiac (heart) muscle itself. This causes hypertrophy or enlargement of the heart, which leads to increased pumping efficiency and consequently a reduction in the resting heart rate.
- It strengthens the respiratory muscles which facilitate the flow of air into and out of the lungs.
- It increases the number of red blood cells to which oxygen binds and hence aids its transportation around the body and to the muscles.
- It improves the efficiency of circulation which helps reduce blood pressure.
- It can help in reducing stress as the exercise triggers a hormonal release which is involved in controlling anxiety and alertness levels.

These factors have been shown to help reduce the risk of cardiovascular disease and hence produce significant health benefits. Consequently, aerobic exercise in a variety of forms has grown in popularity in the non-elite sporting population to maintain health and keep fit.

Training zone

The training zone is the heart rate that needs to be achieved by an athlete for the benefits to the cardiovascular system to be achieved. The individual needs their heart rate to be between 65% and 85% of the maximal heart rate for between 20 and 40 min for a cardiovascular benefit. This needs to occur regularly for these benefits to be maintained and improved further. This should be at least three times per week in the non-elite population.

Maximum heart rate

There are a number of ways to calculate a person's maximum heart rate for training purposes. The simplest way to calculate it and to easily recommend to athletes is as follows:

$$220 - age = \text{Maximum heart rate (beats/min)}$$

For a 30-year-old, the training zone is as follows:

$$220 - 30 = 190 \text{ (max heart rate in beats/min)}$$
$$190 \times 65\% = 123 \text{ beats/min}$$
$$190 \times 85\% = 161 \text{ beats/min}$$

Therefore this athlete needs to keep their heart rate between 123 and 161 beats/min for the duration of the exercise of at least 20 min for a training effect to be achieved.

Aerobic testing

As the conditioning demands on athletes have changed, coaches and conditioners have continued to search for ways to objectively measure fitness so that they can ascertain how an athlete is performing, but also to monitor the effectiveness of their training programmes. If athletes have baseline fitness tests conducted and then they are re-tested, improvements in cardiovascular fitness can be measured.

VO_2 max testing

VO_2 max testing is the gold standard or most accurate test of aerobic or cardiovascular fitness. Its definition is the athlete's maximum capacity to utilise oxygen in a graded exercise test. The testing procedure is not readily available as it requires the athlete's ventilation to be measured very accurately with the concentrations of oxygen and carbon dioxide of inspired and expired air being measured while the athlete performs the graded exercise test on a treadmill or static bike. An athlete's VO_2 max is reached when their oxygen uptake remains constant even though the intensity of the exercise test increases. It is measured in litres/minute (L/min) or millilitres/minute per kilogram (mL/min/kg) of body weight. A score for an elite athlete who participates in an aerobic event such as a rower, long distance runner or cyclist should reach approximately 75 mL/min/kg.

Bleep test

The VO_2 max test is not possible for the majority of athletes, so other tests have been devised to give an objective measure of cardiovascular fitness. The bleep test is perhaps the most common test. It is simply a running-based test which comprises a 20 m shuttle where the athlete has to complete the shuttle inside timed bleeps on a pre-recorded audio tape or CD with the bleeps gradually becoming quicker, thus increasing the intensity of the test. The athlete achieves their score by the level of the test they reach and the number of shuttles in that level. The test goes to Level 21, but an elite athlete should be able to reach at least Level 14 on the test.

TYPES OF AEROBIC TRAINING

Conditioning staff are always looking at developing different training sessions to give the athletes the greatest training benefits. As discussed earlier, it can be in its simplest form maintaining the athlete's heart rate within their training zone for the duration of the session. This is not as effective for elite athletes who need their cardiovascular system to be stressed more vigorously to gain the greatest benefits; therefore other examples will be discussed.

Interval training

Interval training involves the athlete working at near full exertion, i.e. approximately 90% of their maximal heart rate for a period of time, and then interspersed with a rest period of much lower intensity exercise or relative rest. The session is most beneficial when the work to rest ratio is approximately 1 : 1; that is the time of effort is similar to the rest period. As the session progresses, the athlete's recovery will not be complete and their heart rate will not return to its normal resting level. The rest period is often simply a walk back recovery to the starting position or can be a very low intensity continuation of the same exercise. The sessions should be made relevant to the athlete and the demands of their specific event, i.e. running for running-based sports and a rowing session for rowers, etc.

   Examples are as follows:
- Running
  10×400 m with 1 min recovery between each repetition
  12×200 m with 30 s recovery.
- Rowing
  6×500 m ergo with 2 min recovery between reps.
- A pyramid session for ergo or bike
  10 s on, 10 s off
  20 s on, 20 s off
  30 s on, 30 s off
  40 s on, 40 s off
  50 s on, 50 s off
  60 s on, 60 s off
  50 s on, 50 s off
  40 s on, 40 s off
  30 s on, 30 s off
  20 s on, 20 s off
  10 s on, 10 s off

There should be a 2-min rest between sets and repeat three sets. The 'on' period should be with high levels of resistance and at near maximal effort, with the 'off' period at low resistance but continuing the exercise.

Fartlek training

Fartlek training is similar to interval training in that there are periods of high intensity training interspersed with low intensity periods. It is continuous training and therefore is often used by long distance runners as a training method. The session can last for up to 45 min and can, in fact, include anaerobic bursts if it is required in the athlete's event.

   An example of a Fartlek session might be:

- 5 mile run at normal speed
- 8×90 s bursts of increased intensity at 800 m pace with 2–3 min between each increased intensity burst.

Conditioning games

These have become popular training methods in team sports where the athletes play small sided games which are relevant to their sport. The aim is for the athlete to maintain their heart rate at between 75% and 90% of their heart rate maximum for the duration of the game. By keeping the number of team members fairly small, it ensures that all the athletes work maximally for the duration of the game and it is difficult for them not to join in the game and rest.

A good example would be a 3-a-side game of football for 5×5 min periods, or 2-on-2 basketball for 5×3 min periods.

Heart rate monitors

A recent product which has led to further monitoring has been heart rate monitors which are worn by athletes during their sessions and actually record their heart rate throughout a training session.

In this way, their effort levels can be monitored and conditioners and coaches can ensure that their athletes are maintaining their heart rate at the desired levels of towards 85% of the heart rate max for the whole session. It is an accurate way of observing heart rates through a session but also the rate of recovery, which is another good indicator of cardiovascular fitness as this occurs faster in fitter individuals.

ANAEROBIC TRAINING

Anaerobic training is training or exercise where the athlete triggers the metabolism of the glycogen without oxygen present. It occurs in intense exercise which lasts for less than 2 min and is effective in building muscle mass and power. It does, however, lead to the production of waste products such as lactic acid, which is detrimental to muscle function, and therefore, this type of exercise cannot last for longer than 2 min because of the lactic acid build up.

The point where lactic acid builds up in the muscle and circulatory system is termed the *lactic threshold* or *anaerobic threshold* and occurs when the lactic acid is produced more quickly than it can be removed or metabolised. When the lactic threshold is reached, the athlete is unable to continue to perform at the same level and this is often described as 'hitting the wall'. It is, however, possible to train and increase this threshold so that the athlete can perform for longer at the same or greater intensity before the threshold is reached.

For this training effect to occur, the athlete must work maximally and to fatigue. Their recovery period means that as the session progresses, it is just insufficient for the athletes to meet their targets. As long as the athletes continue to put in maximal effort, they will achieve a training effect and improve their lactic threshold. For this to occur, the work to rest ratio needs to be approximately 1:2–4, with the total work time being between 4 and 8 min.

Examples of such sessions are as follows:

- 10×200 m (aim to complete within 30 s) with 90 s recovery
- 5×400 m with 5 min rest
- 10×60 m sprints with 60 s recovery.

Therefore, any event or sport where the athlete is required to work to maximum intensity for periods of up to 2 min needs to include this form of training in their programmes.

STRENGTH TRAINING

Strength training is where different forms of resistance are used to build strength, size and endurance of muscles. It is important for athletes to include strength training in their training programmes, as significant benefits to their function can be achieved, including improved joint function and reduced injury risk given to them by the increased size and strength of the muscles acting over the joints. Weight training is the commonest form of strength training and the principles underpinning it will be discussed further here.

Principles of training

There are different forms of strength training which give rise to different results and improvements in the athlete's performance. It is the differences in the number of repetitions, sets, speed of exercise, weightlift or force required and tempo which cause slightly different adaptations to the muscles and differentiate between the different forms of strength training.

Specificity

It is vital that the exercises which are integrated into each athlete's programme are specific to their individual needs to improve performance in their event. There are now hundreds of exercises that can be tried in the gym which all train the muscles in a slightly different range or different movement pattern.

The strength and conditioning trainers must analyse the movements that occur in the athlete's event and try to replicate these movements in the gym. For example, the squat exercise is very useful when athletes require a sprint or explosive start to running or if jumping is required in their sport.

Also, it has been shown that when training the muscle, the gains are often task- or movement-specific. For example, when strengthening the quadriceps, squat training shows improvements in this form of closed chain knee extension, specifically the squat, but there is no carry over or improvement in open chain knee extension strength. Therefore, it is not just as simple as doing an exercise which uses the muscle group but, importantly, it should be movement- and event-specific for each individual.

Also, not every athlete will require every type of weight training in their programme because the demand of each sport is slightly different. For example, a sprinter will not require endurance training as it is not part of their sport, but of paramount importance is making improvements in power and strength. Likewise, a marathon runner will not need power training and should concentrate on endurance and strength sessions instead.

Strength

For specific strength to be gained the exercise programme must have the following components:

- The weight must be between 75% and 95% of their 1-repetition maximum (1RM) weight
- There should be between 2 and 5 repetitions (reps) in each set of exercises

- There should be between 2 and 5 sets of each exercise
- The session should have between 4 and 10 exercises for the athlete to complete
- The athlete should have between 2 and 5 min of rest between sets
- The speed of exercise should be between 60% and 80% of the maximum speed at which the exercise could be performed
- There should be 2–3 strength sessions per week for up to 6 weeks for strength adaptations to occur.

Power training

Power training is an important component of many athletes' training programmes to provide them with greater force production and at greater speeds. The exercises transfer well to ballistic athletic movements and require good recruitment pattern of the muscles to be effective.

A power session should follow these principles:

- The weight should be moved as quickly as possible through the available range
- 3–5 reps per set
- 3–5 sets
- Work at 40–60% of 1RM
- 3–5 min rest between sets
- A power session needs to be included for at least 6 weeks for advances to be made.

Hypertrophy training

Hypertrophy is where increases in muscle bulk occur. Hypertrophy sessions should follow the following principles:

- 8–15 repetitions per set
- 3–5 sets
- The intensity should be at 60–80% of 1RM
- The rest period between sets should be 1–2 min so that a degree of fatigue occurs.

Endurance training

This component of a training programme requires a far greater number of repetitions and is most commonly used by endurance athletes rather than those who play team sports such as football and rugby.

An endurance session should be based on the following basic principles:

- 25+ reps to fatigue
- 2–3 sets
- 1–2 min rest between sets
- Intensity of 40% of 1RM.

WHAT EQUIPMENT TO USE?

Weight training can be carried out in two main forms. The first adjunct to weight training is by using free weights such as dumbbells and barbells, and second, by weight machines.

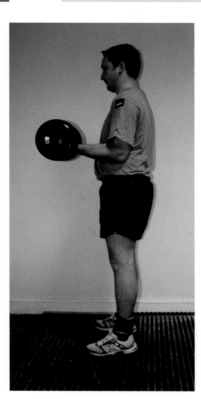

Figure 1.1 Bicep curl.

Free weights

Free weights are where the athlete utilises dumbbells, barbells, medicine balls and other objects to provide the weight or resistance to the exercise. Using free weights allows the athlete to exercise through a full range of movement and perform multijoint exercises. They do, however, require more trunk stability and technique to safely do the exercises. While this can be limiting to novice trainers, it is seen to be a more beneficial training approach for experienced athletes. For examples of exercises using free weights, see the bicep curl in Figure 1.1 and the shoulder press in Figure 1.2.

Weight machines

Weight machines offer a stable base from which exercises can be carried out and are therefore considered to be safer, and thus better for novice weight trainers or athletes recovering initially from injuries. The range of movement is, however, more limited and tends to only allow single joint exercises.

INJURY PREVENTION

As with all areas of training, injuries can occur. It is important with all types of weight and conditioning training that a graduated programme is employed that allows the athlete or individual to adapt to the training gradually.

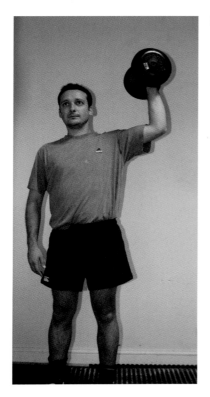

Figure 1.2 Shoulder press.

It is vital that the athlete is taught the correct technique first and that they can reproduce this throughout a training session. Once this has been achieved, they can gradually increase the intensity of the sessions to ensure that they do not sustain an injury. It is only at this point that more rigorous testing can be considered.

Athletes also need to ensure that their training programmes are well planned to ensure that there are adequate rest periods between sessions and that there is sufficient time to train fully before an event or match.

An example of this is the runner who trains for a marathon. Often, individuals decide to do a marathon but do not give themselves sufficient time to build up their training schedule and subsequently suffer overuse injuries.

This is an important consideration for all athletes, regardless of their event, to ensure that the correct technique is implemented and that training programmes are well planned and scheduled.

Chapter | 2 |

Injury prevention

© 2009 Elsevier Ltd, Inc, BV
DOI: 10.1016/B978-0-443-06813-3.00005-3

The ability to prevent an injury is the 'holy grail' of all sports therapists. To reduce the occurrence of an injury and thereby keep the athlete training and competing is the ultimate in excellent care. There are many factors that contribute to achieving this goal and there are many factors that we have no control over that may jeopardise our best efforts; however, one way of identifying which athlete is at risk of what injury, is to perform a screening or profiling medical. This is a top-to-toe musculoskeletal survey of the athlete, taking into consideration their sport, playing position, demands of the sport, their morphology, strength, stature, muscle balance, proprioception, posture, biomechanics, joint range of movement and stability, body control, flexibility and coordination. This is a long list but the process involves progressing through the body, examining each joint and muscle group with the insight of the athlete's past injury history, identifying as you go along any deficiencies, imbalances, structural abnormalities or injuries that would put the athlete at risk of injury. A suggested medical examination protocol is shown in Figure 2.1.

For this process, a list of identified weaknesses can then be addressed by prehabilitation exercises. 'Prehab' exercises to address deficiencies have been shown to reduce injury incidence and are now an integral part of athlete training regimes. There is no fool-proof plan that will keep athletes injury-free but below are some of the essential factors that need to be addressed to succeed.

CORE STABILITY

'Core stability' has been an 'in-vogue' area for sports medics, conditioners and coaches alike. It relates to the musculature around the trunk and pelvis and the move towards ensuring that an athlete has a stable trunk and pelvis which will provide the base for all other movements of the limbs to work from.

It is an area where there is a spectrum as to what it actually means and what should actually occur. Some physiotherapists are at one end and talk about segmental stability of each spinal level, while it tends to be the conditioners who are at the other end of the spectrum and who see it as using all the trunk muscles strongly together to provide the base. In practice, a middle ground needs to be found and both groups of people need to interact and work together to provide the athlete with the best possible programme.

Everyone is in agreement that this stable base around the trunk and pelvis is required to allow the athlete to perform to the best of their ability, but that it is also important to help prevent injuries. It has been shown that instability or excess movements at and around the pelvis can cause compensatory movements to occur at the more distal joints. For example, athletes who have poor gluteal control around their hip and pelvis are unable to control the hip in load-bearing positions, which can cause the hip to internally (medially) rotate. This puts extra

Medical screening/profiling

Date of examination:___/___/___

Name: _____   Date of birth: ___/___/___

Date of last game: ___/___/___   Completed game: Yes / No

Examining doctor: _____   Signature: _____

A.   MEDICAL HISTORY

Significant past medical history

Diabetes	☐	Heart disorder	☐
Epilepsy	☐	Murmurs	☐
Asthma	☐	Palpitations	☐
Heartburn	☐	Ulcer	☐

Other significant medical history: _____

Family history _____   Infectious diseases _____

Smoker: Yes / No   No. per day: _____   Alcohol: Yes / No   Amount per week: _____

Current medications: _____

Current supplements: _____

Preferred NSAID: _____

Allergies: _____

Date of last concussion: ___/___/___

Number of concussions in past 12 months: _____

Other concussion history: _____

Regular strapping: _____

Date of last dental check, mouthguard fitting: _____

B. PLAYING HISTORY and INJURY MANAGERS

Club	Position	Games last 12 months
Treating therapists	Physiotherapist	Doctor

Figure 2.1 Medical examination form.

C. SIGNIFICANT PAST SURGICAL/INJURY HISTORY (including any lost playing time in past 12 months):

Neck : Thoracic : Torso : Lumbar : Sacral

Shoulder : Elbow : Wrists : Hands

Hips : Thighs : Groin : Knees : Shins : Ankles : Feet

D. IMMUNISATION STATUS/BLOOD TESTS

TYPE	YES / NO	DATE OF BOOSTER/TEST
Tetanus		
Polio		
Hepatitis A		
Hepatitis B		
Ferritin	Level: _____	
Hep B abs		
Blood group		

D. PHYSICAL EXAMINATION

Height: _____ cm   Weight: _____ kg   Pulse: _____   PEF: _____

Urinalysis: Glucose _____   Protein _____   Blood _____   Nitrates _____   Bili _____

Visual acuity: Right _____   Left _____ (without glasses)

                                 Right _____   Left _____ (with glasses)

CNS: _____ Fundoscopy _____

CVS: _____

Respiratory: _____

Abdomen: _____

ENT: _____

Cx spine: _____

Thoracic spine: _____

Fingers/thumbs (incl. UCL): _____

Wrists: _____

Marfanoid: Yes / No   Ligamentous hyperlaxity: Yes / No

Standing:

Figure 2.1, cont'd

Posture: _____ Feet: _____ Pelvic symmetry: _____

1 leg squat: (R) _____ (L) _____ Lunge: (R) _____ (L) _____

Gluteal control _____ Trendelenberg _____

Proprioception (R) _____ (L) _____ Hop ¥ 10 (R) _____ (L) _____

Squat _____ Duck walk _____

L/spine: ROM: _____ Quadrant: _____

Ankle dorsiflexion (R) _____ (L) _____

Shoulder

ROM (?arc) Abduction (R) _____ (L) _____

           ER/IR   (R) _____ (L) _____

Scapula ? wasting _____ SHR (R) _____ (L) _____

Rotator cuff power (R) _____ (L) _____

Impingement tests (R) _____ (L) _____
(Neers/Hawkins)

ACJ   Tenderness (R) _____ (L) _____ Scarf test (R) _____ (L) _____

Stability   AP stability (R) _____ (L) _____ Relocation (R) _____ (L) _____

           Apprehension (R) _____ (L) _____ Sulcus (R) _____ (L) _____

Labral tests _____

Other: _____

Spine (supine)

Slump (R) _____ (L) _____ Thomas' (R) _____ (L) _____

Thomas' adductor (R) _____ (L) _____ Flexion (R) _____ (L) _____

SLR (R) _____ (L) _____ Hamstring tightness (R) _____ (L) _____

Leg length _____ Pelvic symmetry _____

Core stability _____ Activating TA: Sit up _____ SLR _____

Hip ROM (IR/ER) (R) _____/_____ (L) _____/_____

      Faber (R) _____ (L) _____ Quadrant (R) _____ (L) _____

Hip flexor strength (R) _____ (L) _____

Adductor tenderness _____ Power _____ Squeeze _____

Figure 2.1, cont'd

Pubic symphysis _____   Inguinal canal _____   Psoas _____

Spine (prone)

L/Sp tenderness _____   L/Sp mobility _____

Facet tenderness _____   SIJ _____

Glut/Ham control & power   (R) _____   (L) _____

Quad length (heel to buttock)   (R) _____   (L) _____

Dial test   (R) _____   (L) _____

Knee

Effusion   (R) _____   (L) _____   PFJ _____

ROM (Ext/flex)   (R) _____ / _____   (L) _____ / _____

Ligaments: MCL   (R) _____   (L) _____   LCL   (R) _____   (L) _____

ACL: Ant draw   (R) _____   (L) _____   Lachman   (R) _____   (L) _____   Pivot   (R) _____   (L) _____

PCL: (R) _____   (L) _____

Joint line: Tenderness   (R) _____   (L) _____   McM   (R) _____   (L) _____   Apley's   (R) _____   (L) _____

Sup tib – fib   (R) _____   (L) _____

Other: _____

Ankle

ROM   TCJ (PF/DF)   (R) _____ / _____   (L) _____ / _____   STJ   (R) _____   (L) _____

Power   (R) _____   (L) _____

Stabilty: Ant draw   (R) _____   (L) _____   Talar tilt   (R) _____   (L) _____

Palpation JLT   (R) _____   (L) _____   Sinus tarsi   (R) _____   (L) _____   Cuboid   (R) _____   (L) _____

5th M/tarsal   (R) _____   (L) _____

Syndesmosis: ER stress   (R) _____   (L) _____   Squeeze   (R) _____   (L) _____

Other: _____

E. GENERAL COMMENTS

_____

_____

_____

_____

_____

Figure 2.1, cont'd

F. RECOMMENDED TREATMENT INTERVENTIONS

_____

_____

_____

_____

_____

_____

_____

G. RECOMMENDED INVESTIGATIONS

_____

_____

_____

_____

_____

_____

Figure 2.1, cont'd

load through the knee with a valgus stress being exerted and hence causing compression to the lateral compartment and stress to the medial ligament. These alignment changes can cause tightness to the iliotibial band and subsequently can cause a lateral tracking of the patella. Further down the chain, it will cause a medial rotation force to the tibia and exert extra load through the medial longitudinal arch of the foot.

An example of this, in the upper limb, can be where poor stability in the lumbar spine leads to protective stiffness developing in the thoracic spine to try and provide the athlete with some stability or rigidity. This stiffness (most commonly limiting extension) leads to excess movement occurring in the shoulder to compensate for the lack of thoracic extension, and is common in athletes who participate in sports that require their shoulder to move repetitively over their head, such as tennis players. This excess movement often leads to instability at the joint or rotator cuff tendinopathies or tears.

Physiotherapists have recently talked about two general groups of muscles: low-load stability muscles and high-level mobility muscles, both of which are discussed below.

 Low-load stability muscles

These muscles, which include the transversus abdominis, multifidus and even the deep parts of psoas, have been discussed as muscles that work at low load and are postural control muscles. They work to provide segmental spinal stability and control and have been shown to have an anticipatory role in controlling the trunk, as they contract before limb movements occur and hence provide the stable base required. However, they have also been shown to lose this anticipatory timing when pain is present and this has been proposed as one reason that low back pain continues and recurs.

Studies have shown that re-training these muscles after an episode of low back pain can reduce the recurrence from about 70% to about 30%. It is therefore an important area for athletes to train to prevent injuries and stop their recurrence.

The exercises in the studies initially tried to isolate a contraction of each muscle and then gradually add load while maintaining the contraction. In practice, more than one of the muscles work at the same time and it is this co-contraction that is effective in maintaining spinal stability. The muscles still need to work and be taught to activate at approximately 30% of maximal contraction but co-contraction is acceptable.

The traditional transversus abdominis exercise is in crook lying and gentle flattening of the low abdomen towards the spine, while breathing. A facilitation technique for those athletes who are struggling with the concept is to use the muscles that stop them from urinating and this can help activate the transversus muscle (Fig. 2.2).

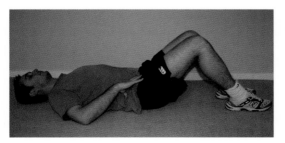

Figure 2.2 Transversus abdominis exercise.

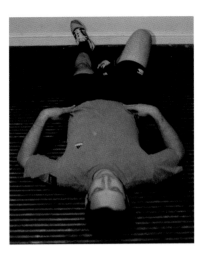

Figure 2.3 Bent knee fallout.

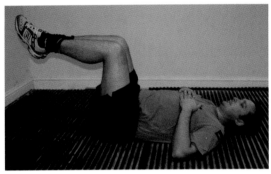

Figure 2.4 Bilateral hip flex.

 ## Floor exercises

All the floor exercises are started in the supine position, with the athlete's knees bent up (crook lying) with lumbar neutral maintained with the activation of the low level core muscles, such as the transversus abdominis.

1. Bent knee fallout
   - The athlete palpates the anterior pelvic bones and slowly rolls alternate knees towards the floor keeping the foot on the floor. The athlete stops when the pelvic control is lost and the opposite pelvic bone rises into their fingers (Fig. 2.3).
2. Unilateral hip flexion
   - The athlete has their hands under the lumbar spine to monitor the movement and slowly lifts and lowers alternate knees towards the chest. He/she stops and lowers if lumbar neutral is lost by either excessive pressure or a pressure loss felt through their hands under their lumbar spine. The exercise is progressed to flexing both hips and bringing both knees up towards the chest and then lowering again (Fig. 2.4).
3. Unilateral hip and knee extension
   - The athlete starts with both feet lifted off the floor at a 90° hip flex. The athlete then extends one hip so the foot is an inch off the floor and then extends the knee until the point where lumbar neutral is lost. The progression is to do this with both legs together (Fig. 2.5).

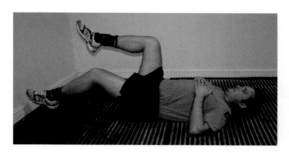

Figure 2.5 Unilateral hip and knee extension.

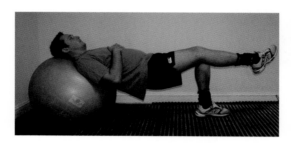

Figure 2.6 Single leg extension.

The floor exercises can be progressed and a gym ball can be used to make the core stability exercises more difficult and interesting for the athlete. The athlete needs to activate the transversus abdominus and other stability muscles while performing these exercises.

High-level mobility muscles

The main function of stronger muscles of the trunk such as the rectus abdominis, erector spinae and oblique muscles is to move the trunk. However, in many athletes who have a poor low-level core, these muscles are also used to produce stability or rigidity through an isometric type contraction. It is difficult for the muscles to do two jobs at the same time which are at opposite ends of the spectrum. They cannot stabilise isometrically on one hand and then cause movement through a concentric contraction on the other, and therefore athletes must be able to activate the deeper stability muscle as well. However, these mobiliser muscles are needed when greater loads are exerted to the body and to contribute to the stability of the spine through their contraction as the stability muscles cannot cope on their own. This co-contraction is vital to prevent injuries and allow a stable platform for the limbs to work from in high demand and loading sports.

Examples of low-load floor-based exercises with progressions to gym ball exercises and finally to higher-load core exercises follow.

 Gym ball exercises

1. Single leg extensions
   - The athlete lies with the shoulder blades on the ball, feet on the floor and the buttocks raised, so the lumbar spine is in neutral. The athlete then extends one knee to lift the foot off the floor and holds the position (Fig. 2.6).

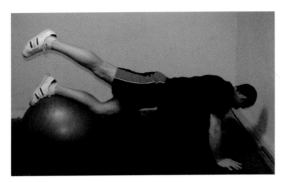

Figure 2.7 Prone hip extension.

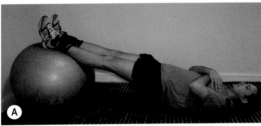

Figure 2.8 (A) Supine hip extension. (B) Supine hip extension with one leg lifted off the ball.

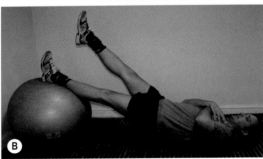

2. Prone hip extensions
- The athlete is in a prone position with hands on the floor and feet or shins on the ball. One foot is then lifted off the ball and lumbar neutral is again maintained (Fig. 2.7).

3. Supine hip extension
- The athlete lies supine with the feet resting on the ball. He then lifts his buttocks off the floor by pressing through his heels (Fig. 2.8A). This can be made more difficult by then lifting one leg off the ball (Fig. 2.8B).

Higher-level exercise

1. Plank
- The athlete is prone with his elbows under his shoulders. He lifts his pelvis off the floor so he is resting on his elbows and toes only. Load can be added to his back to make the exercise more difficult through free weights (Fig. 2.9).

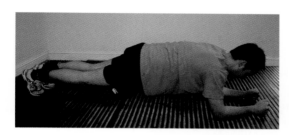

Figure 2.9 Plank.

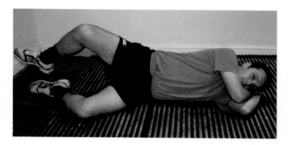

Figure 2.10 The clam.

2. Traditional sit-ups and their many variations will train the high-level muscles in small movement but will also help strengthen them for their control role as well.

Another vital part of trunk and pelvic stability are the gluteal muscles. While the gluteal muscles are important in producing movements of the hip joint, they are also responsible for providing stability to the sacroiliac joint and vital in controlling the rotation of the hip in weight-bearing positions. It is their role in maintaining a neutrally rotated hip which is vital in providing the stable base for the lower limb to function from. It is most often a lack of lateral rotation control which causes problems in the lower limb and there are, therefore, some useful gluteal strengthening exercises, which are highlighted below.

Gluteal muscle (glutes) exercises

1. The clam
   • Sidelying, the hips and knees are flexed to 90°, the top knee is lifted up using the glutes and keeping the heels together
   • This can be progressed to lifting the top leg up so that the heels are also apart (Fig. 2.10).
2. Glutes, standing at wall
   • The athlete stands side-on to the wall with the hip nearest the wall flexed to 90°. The hip is pushed into the wall while the standing hip is externally rotated, with the standing leg being the glute that is working (Fig. 2.11).
3. Hip extension/abductions in sidelying
   • Sidelying, the athlete starts with the upper hip flexed and adducted slightly across the body. The exercise is to quickly extend and abduct the hip up and behind, and then return back to the starting position (Fig. 2.12).

With the stable platform provided by good co-contraction of all of the above muscles, the athlete is less likely to sustain overuse injuries which are commonly triggered by poor movement patterns and excess load being transferred to the

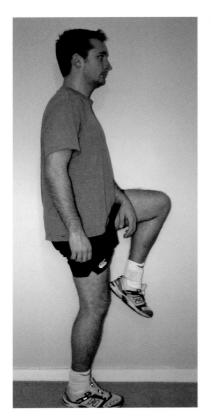

Figure 2.11 Glutes in standing at wall.

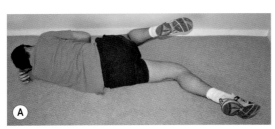

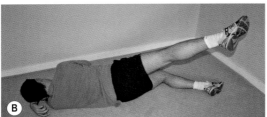

Figure 2.12 (A,B) Hip extension.

tendon or muscle. These exercises are therefore vital to every athlete, to prevent missing valuable playing time.

PROPRIOCEPTION OR BALANCE EXERCISES

The term 'proprioception' is simply the body's understanding of a joint's position in space. It equates to an athlete's ability to control their movements and correct the position of their joints during these movements. It is a vital physiological characteristic for successful participation in sport.

The brain receives feedback from mechanoreceptors and nerve endings in and around the joints as they move, which then allows small compensatory movements to occur that maintain or return the athlete's joint to its normal alignment. These small movements occur very quickly and prevent a joint moving to an extreme end-of-range position where damage can occur to the passive restraints, such as the ligaments, joint capsule and active restraints, such as the muscles acting over the joint.

Consequently, this is an area which athletes need to be very aware of to improve performance and prevent injuries. It is an area that can be trained with improvements often equating to a reduction in ligament injuries. The athlete must also have a good strength base in the muscles acting over the joint, because it is the control of these muscles that produce the small righting movements. Therefore, a proprioceptive programme needs to be integrated into a strength programme.

Two of the most common areas where proprioceptive rehabilitation or 'prehabilitation' occurs are in the lower limb and the shoulder.

The lower limb

The joints of the ankle and knee are particularly susceptible to ligament injury and proprioceptive training can be very useful in preventing or rehabilitating from these injuries.

The exercises need to be functional and need to be weight-bearing or in a closed kinetic chain.

An example of a proprioceptive programme with a progression of exercises is given below:

1. Single-leg standing ×30 s (Fig. 2.13)
    *   Make more difficult by:
        ■ standing on an uneven or softer surface, e.g. pillow, rolled-up towels
        ■ standing, passing and catching a ball
        ■ do functional movements for their sport, e.g. hitting a ball against a wall.
2. Single-leg standing with eyes closed ×30 s (Fig. 2.14)
    *   The exercise can be made more difficult in the same way as above in single-leg standing.
3. Forward hop onto one leg and hold ×10 s.
4. Sideways hop onto one leg and hold ×10 s.
5. Grid hops, e.g. set out a numbered grid and the athlete must hop on one leg to the different numbers.
6. Single-leg squats (Fig. 2.15)
    *   Make more difficult by:
        ■ being up on toes
        ■ being on an unstable surface, such as a pillow.

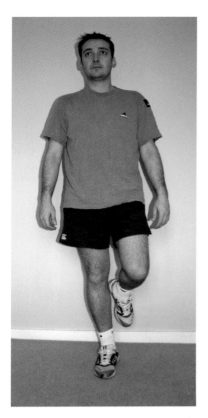

Figure 2.13 Single-leg standing.

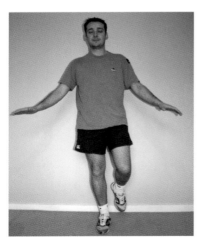

Figure 2.14 Single-leg standing with eyes closed.

7. Wobbleboard or BOSU balance
   - Progress as above:
     - Single-leg standing ×30 s (Fig. 2.16)
     - Single-leg standing with eyes closed ×30 s
     - Forward hop onto one leg and hold ×10 s (Fig. 2.17)

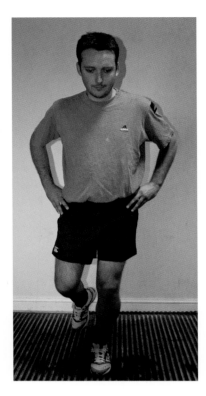

Figure 2.15 Single-leg squat.

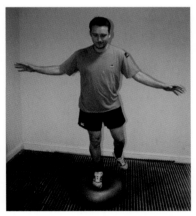

Figure 2.16 Single-leg BOSU balance.

- Lateral (sideways) hop onto one leg and hold ×10 s (Fig. 2.18)
- Single-leg squats.

Other exercises that reproduce functional movement patterns but also involve a strength component can be very useful and can be combined with the specific proprioceptive exercises. Some examples:

Knee drives

The athlete stands on one leg, with the other leg behind in a lunge-type position. He drives his leg through and up in a running motion, and then backwards again

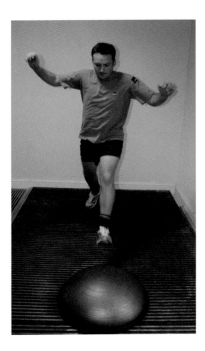

Figure 2.17 Forward BOSU hop.

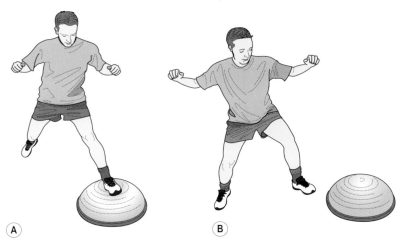

(A)   (B)

Figure 2.18 Lateral hop.

at a fast pace. This can be repeated starting with 10 repetitions and building up to sets of 25 or 30 in elite athletes (Fig. 2.19).

Walk-through lunges

The athlete does a lunge, then drives up to stand on the front leg and pauses for 2 s to test their balance before lunging forward onto the other leg. It should be a dynamic movement pattern. This should start with 5 repetitions and build up to 20 repetitions in the elite (Fig. 2.20).

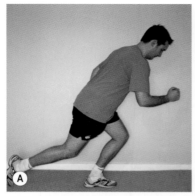

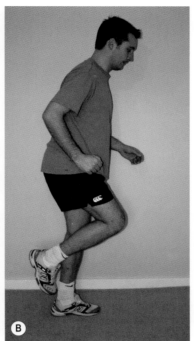

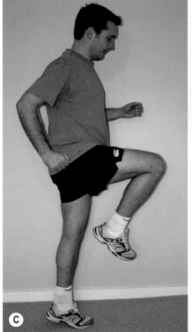

Figure 2.19 (A,B,C) Knee drive.

Figure 2.20 Walk-through lunge.

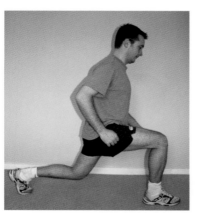

Jump lunges

The athlete starts in a lunge position. He then jumps straight up in the air and swaps legs over, so the other leg is now in front. This is repeated without pausing between repetitions. Again a starting point would be 5 repetitions and building up to at least 20 in elite athletes.

Shoulder and upper limb

The shoulder has the greatest available range of any joint and is involved in all sporting activities, whether it is simply in running or more complex actions such as throwing or in racquet sports.

It is therefore at risk of injury when it is taken through its wide range of motion, often at great speed and hence having significant forces being exerted on the joint and the surrounding soft tissues.

It is very important to aid an athlete's proprioception around the joint to prevent injuries, and again combine this with strengthening work.

A sample of exercises is shown below:

1. Single-arm ball movements on wall
   - In a figure-of-8 pattern or in a cross-pattern (Fig. 2.21)
   - In different positions, e.g. full flexion, 90° abduction/lateral rotation, full horizontal flexion.
2. Ball catching in supine with shoulder in abduction/lateral rotation (Fig. 2.22)
   - Start with a light ball and progress to catching medicine balls of increasing weight
   - Make more difficult by closing the eyes.
3. Theraband rotation catches
   - From an abduction/lateral rotation starting point, the athlete does a quick medial rotation movement and then catches the movement against the band and slowly returns the shoulder to the starting point.
4. Press-ups on a wobbleboard, BOSU ball or sit-fit cushion (Fig. 2.23)
   - Progress to single-armed press-ups.

TAPING

Various taping techniques have been developed by physiotherapists to try to support and protect joints. Taping tends to be used for three main reasons:

1. It is commonly used after injury to protect a joint which has increased laxity after a ligament sprain. It attempts to prevent excess movement and support the previously injured ligament and therefore will be tightly placed directly over and along the course of the ligament.
2. It is used to try to prevent common injuries. This is common practice in North American sports, such as American football where every player has both ankles strapped for every session to try to prevent ligament sprains.
3. For confidence or added proprioception. A player may have had a long-standing injury or feel weak at a specific joint, and when the tape is applied tightly to the skin, it can provide added proprioceptive feedback and the feeling of added stability which may give the athlete added confidence in the joint.

In practice, the effectiveness of the tape to actually prevent excess movement may not last much more than 15 min or so, depending on how well the tape has been applied and how intense the sporting activity has been and hence how loose

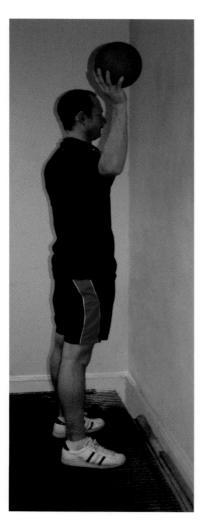

Figure 2.21 Single-arm ball movements on wall.

the tape has become. However, the proprioceptive benefits of the tape may last for as long as the tape remains *in situ* and it therefore can be a very useful technique for protecting joints or preventing injuries.

Some useful examples of taping are shown below.

- Ankle: lateral ligaments
- Knee: medial collateral ligament
- Shoulder: to stop lateral rotation and aid proprioception.

 WARM-UP

Warm-ups are an integral part of the preparation of any athlete for their sport and have been for many years. However, they have been an ever-evolving and changeable part of an athlete's preparation as conditioners and coaches try to find the most effective manner to ready the athlete.

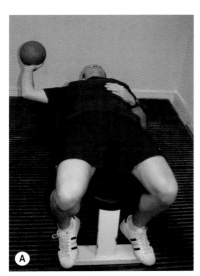

Figure 2.22 (A,B) Ball catching in supine with shoulder in abduction.

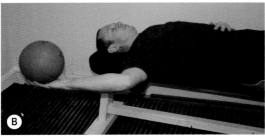

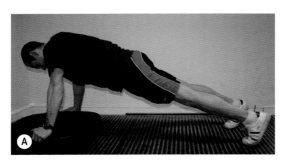

Figure 2.23 (A,B) BOSU press-up.

The warm-up is an essential component for a number of reasons:

1. To prepare the athlete's body for the activity in which they are about to take part
2. To practise some of the key areas of the athlete's sport or activity
3. To mentally prepare the athlete by carrying out some of the sport or activity-specific drills
4. To try to prevent injuries.

 ## Physical elements

The warm-up needs to comprise a number of elements that will gradually replicate many of the movements the athlete will be required to do.

First, there must be a cardiovascular element where the heart rate increases and blood is pumped into all the muscles which will be used in the sport.

Second, the muscles must be prepared for the strain they are about to be put under and consequently a stretching programme must be included. As discussed previously, a dynamic stretching regime is best for preparing the athlete to perform at their best and hence, this must be included and be an integral part of the warm-up.

It is still possible for athletes to do some static stretching but this must take place at the very start of their warm-up and then be followed by a dynamic stretching programme. This static stretching may help some athletes mentally begin their preparation and give some minimal length changes before the muscles are activated in a dynamic and more functional manner thereafter. If athletes have been doing static stretching for a number of years, it can be an important psychological factor in their own preparation and as long as there is a dynamic component that follows the static stretch, performance will not be impeded.

Third, functional movements and sport-specific movements should be included to stimulate the neuromuscular system in readiness for the activity. This might be the serve in tennis, or passing a ball over varied distances in rugby or football or bowling in cricket.

In all the above areas, the movements need to be gradually progressed in range and intensity until the player gets to full range or speed, so that their body is fully prepared.

It is hoped therefore that this preparation will mean that injuries are less likely to occur because the body is in a state of readiness and has already carried out the majority of stressful movement patterns in a graduated way before the high intensity of the game or race begins.

Sport-specific and mental elements

By including sport-specific drills, it not only allows the body to prepare physically but also allows the athlete to prepare mentally. The athlete should start to go through the movements and activities that they are about to do to allow them to 'switch-on' to the game or race.

This should start with simple drills as the athlete begins and then can become more complex towards the end of the warm-up as the body becomes better prepared physically and the intensity rises.

 ## STRETCHING

Stretching has been one of the most commonly discussed and debated topics among sports medics and conditioners in recent times. The debate has raged about the differences between static and dynamic stretching and where and when they should be incorporated into a sportsperson's training programme.

They are both in fact very important and therefore need to be included in every sportsperson's training programme. The differences will be discussed here and a suggested programme with examples will also be proposed.

Static stretching

Static stretching is simply where a muscle is taken to its fully lengthened position and held for a period of time. It has been the mainstay of warm-ups for many years, although there is now a trend away from using it. This is due to the fact that there has been much debate as to whether the use of static stretching is in fact detrimental to performance when used as part of a warm-up. Some studies have concluded that the use of static stretching before sprinting and jumping produces a negative effect on performance and therefore should no longer be used. However, the majority of these studies have compared static stretching to dynamic stretching in a warm-up and found that dynamic stretching simply produces a better performance outcome than a purely static stretch warm-up. When you look further into the research, however, there have been very few studies that have fully investigated a combined approach where both static and dynamic stretching are used. To counter this, there have in fact been other studies which have found no significant difference between the approaches, so this is an area which will be discussed further in the warm-up section.

Static stretching remains an important component in injury prevention, as studies have shown that players with reduced muscle length (commonly this has been the hamstrings) are more likely to sustain a muscle strain.

Muscle tightness can also cause load to be transferred elsewhere in the body, with injuries occurring there instead and this is common in the lumbar spine. Players with tight hamstrings or hip flexors will often transfer load and strain to their lumbar spine where excessive compensatory movements then take place and subsequent dysfunctions occur.

Therefore, when taking into account these two factors, it is important that a player's muscle length is screened regularly and that they are given programmes to address any reductions in muscle length.

Static stretching has been shown to be more effective than dynamic stretching in improving muscle length and should therefore be used to elicit these changes.

Duration of static stretching

Muscles

Again, there has been a widely debated topic as to the time it actually takes for adaptations to occur and muscle length to change.

For significant changes to occur to a muscle's length, the stretch must be sustained for between 20 and 30 seconds, repeated a number of times and then continued over a period of weeks.

It would therefore be our suggestion that a stretching programme involves each stretch lasting 30 s, being repeated 5 times, and that it is carried out at least twice a day over a month-long period for significant changes to be noticed.

Tendons

As tendons have a far greater percentage of collagen and hence are a more rigid structure, it will take significantly longer for differences to occur here. This is an important consideration when tendons have been injured, such as after an Achilles rupture or ankle injury, where a period of immobilisation has occurred and the tendon has become shortened.

Stretches here must be sustained for at least 2 min with 3 repetitions and carried out at least twice a day for a 'creep' effect to occur on the collagenous tissue. This again may take a significant number of weeks for an effect to be noticed.

Some good examples of static stretches are detailed below:

1. Gastrocnemius stretch
   - Press-up type position, push heel to floor keeping the knee straight (Fig. 2.24).
2. Achilles or soleus muscle stretch
   - Standing facing the wall, keep heel on the floor and bend the knee. It is important to keep the knee positioned over the second toe so that the medial longitudinal arch of the foot does not collapse and a true Achilles stretch is achieved (Fig. 2.25).
3. Hamstring stretch
   - Lying supine, hold behind the knee, and then straighten the knee (Fig. 2.26). This eliminates any lumbar spine flexion movement and localises the stretch to the hamstring.

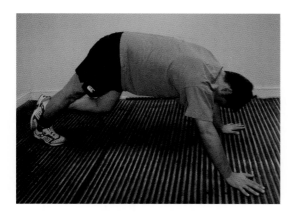

Figure 2.24
Gastrocnemius stretch.

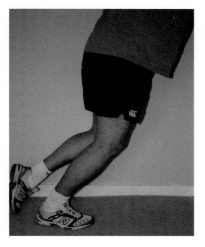

Figure 2.25 Soleus stretch.

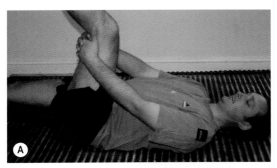

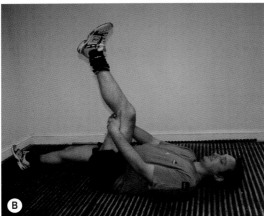

Figure 2.26 (A,B) Hamstring stretch.

4. Quadriceps
   - Lying prone, pull heel to buttock again helping to try and maintain a more lumbar neutral position and try to prevent excessive lumbar extension (Fig. 2.27).
5. Hip flexors
   - Half-kneeling, first posteriorly rotate the pelvis to fix the lumbar spine in neutral and prevent lumbar extension, and then push the hips forward until a stretch is elicited in the back leg (Fig. 2.28).
6. Glutes
   - In crook lying, rest one foot on the other bent knee and pull the knee and hip into adduction to achieve the stretch (Fig. 2.29).
   - Alternatively, in prone on elbows, bring one knee up into hip and knee flexion under the body and again adduct to achieve the stretch.
7. Adductors
   - Standing, simply widen the stance and lean to one side over the knee, keeping both feet on the floor to achieve the adductor stretch.
   - Alternatively, sitting, bring the heels towards the groin and then push both knees together down towards the floor (Fig. 2.30).
8. Lumbar spine
   - Lying supine, bend one knee up and then roll it over to the other side of the body and rest it onto the floor. There will be a tendency for the shoulder on the same side of the body to lift up so the stretch is made greater by keeping both shoulders flat to the floor (Fig. 2.31).

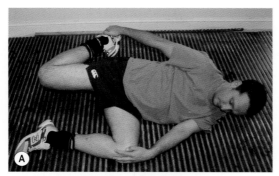

Figure 2.27 (A,B) Quad stretch.

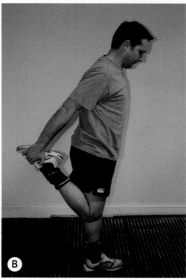

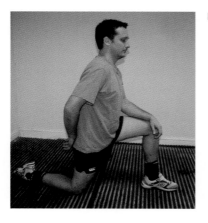

Figure 2.28 Hip flexor stretch.

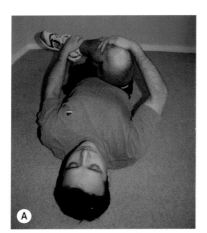

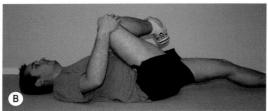

Figure 2.29 (A,B) Glutes stretch.

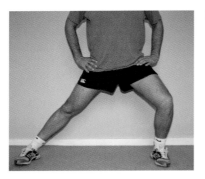

Figure 2.30 Adductor stretch.

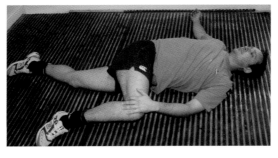

Figure 2.31 Lumbar stretch.

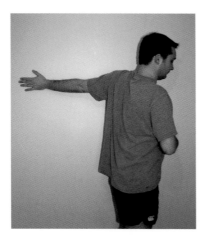

Figure 2.32 Pectoral stretch.

9. Thoracic spine
   - Sitting, so the pelvis is fixed, rotate the upper body and hold.
10. Pectorals
   - The pectorals should be stretched in two positions to stretch the two parts of the muscle.
   - First, the elbow should be fully extended and the shoulder raised to 90° flexion. It should then be horizontally extended behind the athlete. This is for the sternal head of the muscle (Fig. 2.32).
   - For the clavicular head, the shoulder should be flexed to 130° and then extended once more.
11. Triceps
   - With the shoulder full flexed above the head, flex the elbow behind the head and use the other hand to take the shoulder into full range flexion while maintaining full elbow flexion (Fig. 2.33).
12. Cervical spine
   - The normal movements and particularly rotation and side flexion should be used for cervical stretching. The isolated cervical movement should be used and held passively with the hand as shown below.

Hold–relax stretch technique

This is a technique which can be very beneficial to increase muscle length and, consequently, the range of movement.

The athlete requires a partner to achieve this technique as it requires a purely passive stretch to occur after the hold or activation component. The muscle is initially taken passively to its end of range or stretched position and then it is activated against the resistance of the stretching partner, although the activation of the muscle should not actually cause any movement at the joint in which the muscle acts over. This active movement should be held for 7 s before the athlete's stretch partner takes the joint, and hence the muscle, further into its available range. The passive stretch component still needs to be held for 20–30 s before the activation occurs again. This technique can be repeated 3–5 times with excellent increase in range possible.

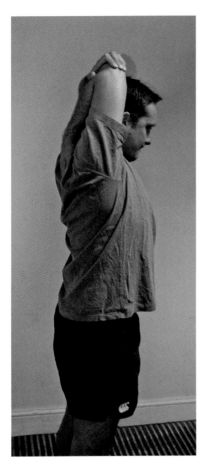

Figure 2.33 Tricep stretch.

 Dynamic stretching

Dynamic stretching has become the warm-up technique of choice over the past few years, with conditioners teaching and athletes hence using the techniques to prepare themselves for their sport.

Simply, dynamic stretching is where the muscles and the joints that they act over are taken actively through their available range without holding the position for any length of time.

Studies have shown that dynamic stretching allows athletes to improve their performance in athletic tasks such as sprinting and jumping when they have prepared using these techniques. It is thought that the dynamic movements help prepare a muscle for activity by replicating the functional movement patterns which are to be carried out in the sport, together with having a neuromuscular effect of stimulating the stretch reflex of the muscle–tendon units.

Dynamic stretching exercises have, however, been shown to be less beneficial in providing long-term changes in actual muscle length, so their inclusion in training programmes should be restricted to the warm-up components of athletes' training.

Repetitions

The dynamic stretch should start gently and then be repeated a number of times with a gradual increase in the range of movement each time until the athlete is moving through the full available range.

1. Hamstrings
   - Leg swings
   - Hurdles
   - Forward leans.
2. Hip flexors and quads
   - Lunges.
3. Adductors
   - Hips up and out.
4. Glutes
   - Cross one knee over the other and forward lean.
5. Calves
   - Press-up position, push calves down to floor then back up onto toes
   - Bent knee walks.
6. Lumbar spine
   - Lumbar rotations.
7. Thoracic spine
   - Thoracic rotations.
8. Shoulders
   - Shoulder swings forward and back
   - Pecs in horizontal flexion.

PROTECTIVE EQUIPMENT

Many sports now allow players to use various pieces of protective clothing or equipment to help prevent injuries.

These differ substantially between each sport and it is therefore very important for each individual sportsperson to check the rules and regulations for their own sport to ascertain what is allowed by each governing body.

These pieces of equipment may be mandatory or their use can be at the discretion of each individual.

However, as technology improves and more money is invested into these areas, it can provide athletes with an important way of trying to prevent injuries.

Some common sports and common pieces of equipment are listed in Box 2.1.

Box 2.1 **Sports equipment**				
Cricket	*Rugby*	*Football*	*Squash*	*Hockey*
Box	Gumshield	Gumshield	Eye protectors	Gumshield
Helmet	Shoulder pads	Shin pads		Shin pads
Pads	Shin pads			Gloves
Gloves				Helmet and
Thigh pad				pads for
Forearm pad				goalkeepers

COOL-DOWN

A cool-down is carried out at the end of a sporting activity and is used to try to limit the degree of delayed onset muscle soreness (DOMS) suffered by an athlete and hence promote recovery. It is also often an ideal time for an athlete to restore or even gain muscle length via a static stretching session, as the muscles are warm and therefore more pliable.

There should be two main components to a cool-down:

1. Light cardiovascular (CV) component
    -   Light CV activity is beneficial to cause the muscles to contract at a low level and work as a muscle pump to remove the waste products of exercise such as lactic acid.
    -   This can be carried out through light jogging, cycling or swimming. Swimming or jogging in water can be particularly useful as it utilises the hydrostatic pressure or compressive forces of the water to aid the muscle pump and remove the waste products.
2. Stretching
    -   A light static stretch should also be included in a cool-down to restore or even increase muscle length after exercise.
    -   The static stretches should again be held for between 20 and 30 s and repeated at least 3–5 times for each muscle group for maximum benefit.

If these components are carried out, they can limit the amount of DOMS and hence promote a faster recovery and facilitate an earlier return to full training.

When *not* to do a cool-down

An athlete who has sustained an injury should not carry out a full cool-down. The injury can either be a muscle strain, muscle haematoma or even a joint strain, and the exercise will increase the blood flow to the affected area. As the first part of the inflammatory process begins with the injury and the associated bleeding, the increased blood flow to the area can cause further bleeding and make the injury worse. Thus, the injured area should be rested, but unaffected areas can still be stretched.

RECOVERY

There has also been a great deal of interest in developing other post-exercise recovery strategies which can be used to minimise post-exercise muscle soreness, control any bleeding that could occur and hence limit the degree of any minor injury that may have been sustained.

Recovery strategies include:

Ice baths

-   The athlete immerses their body into ice cold water, which can be as low as 5° Celsius, which causes a vasoconstriction or narrowing effect on the blood vessels.
-   This narrowing effect can be beneficial in limiting bleeding as it decreases the blood flow to the affected area.

- It is also useful to reduce DOMS when it is combined with a contrast of heat, via a hot bath or shower (which causes vasodilation or opening of the blood vessels). This closing and then opening of the blood vessels is thought to aid the flushing effect and removal of the waste products (lactic acid) from the muscles after exercise.
- There are still a limited number of studies which have shown definitive evidence as to the positive effects or ideal time of immersion. However, anecdotal evidence from a wide variety of athletes has shown significant perceived benefits from their use and therefore they should be recommended to athletes as part of their recovery programme.

Timings

There is no definitive research as yet to give an ideal time for immersion in the ice baths. However, two beneficial protocols are as follows:

- 1 min ice: 1 min heat ×5 repetitions
- 3 min ice: 3 min heat ×2–3 repetitions.

It is worth the athlete trialling different time variations and finding out which protocol provides the greatest benefit for them as it remains a relatively subjective recovery technique thus far.

Massage

Light massage techniques which encourage movement of fluid such as effleurage can be useful to aid in the removal of post-exercise waste products. However, it is important that there is no soft tissue injury present as massage increases the blood flow to the area and, therefore, could cause extra bleeding to occur if it is carried out to the injured area immediately after the injury has been sustained.

It is suggested, therefore, that massage does not occur immediately post-match and for a further 16 h in athletes who have been participating in a contact sporting activity, to ensure that the athlete has not sustained a muscle haematoma or bruise.

Chapter | 3 |

Nutrition

© 2009 Elsevier Ltd, Inc, BV
DOI: 10.1016/B978-0-443-06813-3.00006-5

ENERGY FOR EXERCISE

We all need energy for exercise. Energy is the basic requirement for any form of activity.

It comes from the food we eat and fluids we drink but how much is enough? Too little and we run the risk of under-performing and getting fatigued, too much and we gain weight. What form of exercise we perform also plays a role. Whether we are involved in endurance or explosive activities or whether we are watching our weight, or male or female, we all need energy to exercise but the balance of that energy requirement varies from one to the other.

How quickly we need that energy is also a factor. If we need the energy over a 20 s sprint, then it has to be quickly and freely available as opposed to the slow drip feed supply of a marathon runner. Where that energy is stored and available is important and this reflects the form of energy we take in.

Energy production

The unit of energy is ATP (adenosine triphosphate) which when broken down releases energy. There are three systems of releasing energy from ATP which work together to provide the energy requirement depending on what exercise regime is being followed.[1]

1. ATP-CP
   - ATP is linked with creatine phosphate (CP) as a small store in muscles readily available for fast activity. It is used for short sharp explosive activity and only lasts 5–7 s before the muscle store is depleted. This system is used for sprinting where the energy is needed instantly and therefore does not require oxygen nor distant stores of ATP that would take too long to get to the muscle (Fig. 3.1).
2. Anaerobic energy
   - This provides 100 s of power-based energy. This system produces more energy than the ATP-CP system, and for longer, but is still too quick for oxygen to be involved. In the ATP-CP system, energy is instantly available but here it requires glucose to be broken down to ATP and lactic acid, releasing the ATP for energy. The by-product, lactic acid, can result in muscle cramps and so is not the most efficient energy system for, e.g. a 400 m runner (Fig. 3.2).
3. Aerobic energy
   - This is a slower, more efficient, system of producing ATP and releases 20 times the amount of ATP than the anaerobic system. Glucose is broken down with oxygen to produce the majority of ATP but fat can also be used to produce ATP. This is what happens with training where fat is used preferentially thus conserving the glucose/glycogen stores and reducing the chances of glucose deficiency that happens when an endurance runner 'hits the wall'. Protein is also a source of ATP but not

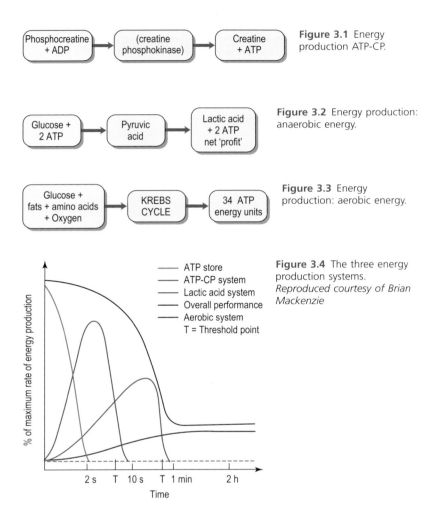

Figure 3.1 Energy production ATP-CP.

Figure 3.2 Energy production: anaerobic energy.

Figure 3.3 Energy production: aerobic energy.

Figure 3.4 The three energy production systems. *Reproduced courtesy of Brian Mackenzie*

as efficient as when glucose is metabolised, e.g. in the long-distance runner (Fig. 3.3).

Some athletic events require purely one energy system to be utilised but most require a combination of all three (Fig. 3.4). Training fine tunes the efficiency of each system appropriate to the event which is being trained for.

Energy values

Energy in the form of ATP is derived from carbohydrates (glucose), fats and proteins but which energy system is used is determined by the following factors:

- Type of activity performed
- Intensity of activity
- Duration of activity
- Frequency of activity
- Fitness level of the athlete
- Diet of the athlete.

If you intensify the level of activity then the body transfers from a fat source to a glucose source of energy. However, the longer you exercise, more fat is metabolised in preference to glucose in an attempt to conserve the limited supply of glucose within the muscles and liver. The balance of fat and glucose, therefore, depends on the exercise training you are undertaking. A sprinter has no need for fat as a store, as his event is over very quickly. They will therefore have very little lean body fat, whereas a marathon runner, although thin, may need fat as a source of energy, as will a swimmer who may benefit from some fat to act as buoyancy. Therefore, rather than looking at the weight of an athlete, we should be measuring the percentage body fat and muscle mass as a true measure of how well we are shaping up to our energy needs.

Energy intake

So how much is right? If we take in too much carbohydrate or protein, then the excess is stored as glycogen and the protein is excreted. Taking in too much fat means that this will be stored within the body. To reduce the body fat we need to reduce the intake and increase the fat burning activity in the form of longer durations of exercise. To increase the protein in lean muscle mass we need to increase the protein and carbohydrate in our diet and increase our exercise and resistance exercise regimes.

Take home points

- Tailor your energy intake to your exercise needs.
- Not all the fat in your diet is bad.
- Muscle mass and percentage lean body fat are better measures than body weight.
- Fatigue may be dietary in origin, not just as a result of over-training.

INGREDIENTS FOR ENERGY

The different types of energy sources and their sub-divisions can be confusing and distracting. The three sources of energy are as follows[2]:

1. Carbohydrates
    - Essentially, this is glucose which is stored as glycogen in muscles and the liver. Carbohydrates exist in our diet in two forms:
      a. Sugars (mono or disaccharides): sugar, fruits, honey, vegetables, sugar cane
      b. Starches (polysaccharides): these are larger molecules which take the body more time to break down and release the glucose, e.g. pasta, potatoes (Fig. 3.5).
    - It is not always helpful to describe foods as simple or complex carbohydrates, as often foods contain a mixture of different types.
2. Proteins
    - These are the building blocks for life. The units for protein, the amino acids, are stored in muscles where there is a limited capacity and any excess is either stored as fat or carbohydrate.
    - Amino acids are divided into those essential ones (which are found in all animal sources of proteins) and the semi-essential and non-essential ones.

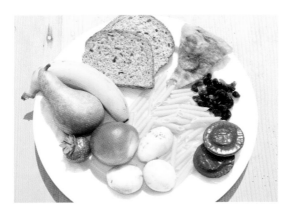

Figure 3.5
Carbohydrates.

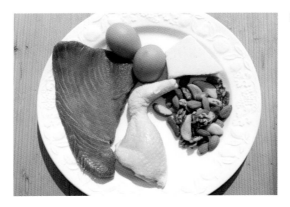

Figure 3.6 Proteins.

- Protein rich foods include:
  - Milk
  - Yoghurt
  - Fish (especially tuna and salmon)
  - Eggs (boiled, scrambled or in omelettes)
  - Meat (beef, lamb, ham)
  - Poultry (chicken)
  - Grains and nuts, especially muesli (Fig. 3.6).
- Proteins are also the building blocks for increasing muscle size and are therefore essential dietary components for those athletes wishing to gain muscle bulk or strength from weight training or resistance exercise.
3. Fats
   - These are essential as a fuel for endurance training, and consist of fatty acids and vitamins A, D, E and K. It is important not to avoid all fats, as the body will use other sources as an energy source, such as carbohydrate, resulting in residual fatigue when the body's store of carbohydrate is so low that fatigue and lethargy result.
   - Fats are divided into saturated and unsaturated (mono-unsaturated and poly-unsaturated) fats. It is important to avoid saturated fats and enhance the unsaturated ones as these reduce the total cholesterol and LDL-cholesterol levels that are harmful in atherosclerosis and heart disease.

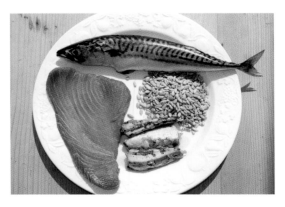

Figure 3.7 Fats.

- Fats are also a source of essential fatty acids in the form of omega-3 (salmon, tuna, mackerel, linseeds and soya bean oil) and omega-6 (sunflower seeds and oil, and nuts). Omega-3 food sources are also the most 'protective' against heart disease (Fig. 3.7).

Take home points

- Eat a variety of foods and enjoy what you eat.
- Eat more carbohydrates, especially cereals and starchy foods.
- Don't be afraid of fats but choose unsaturated ones.
- Eat moderate protein – more is not better and oily fish is best.

Carbohydrates

Glucose is stored in the form of glycogen in muscles and in the liver and is the preferred and most efficient source of energy. Glycogen stores are relatively small and run out after a few days of exercise if not replenished. The amount needed to be re-stocked depends on the exercise regime that is being followed.

The bulk of carbohydrate should come from cereals or starchy food sources such as:

- Bread
- Potatoes
- Rice
- Pasta
- Cereals.

The remainder is gained from sugar, fruits and juices.

You should tailor your intake to your energy expenditure, so if you have a high daily load of intensive exercise you should have an equally high carbohydrate intake, with regular snacks in-between feeds.

The speed with which the glucose is absorbed into the blood stream and hence its availability as a substrate for energy release is also a factor in your choice of carbohydrate foods. The glycaemic index (GI)[3] is a measure of this. Highly absorbed carbohydrates have a high GI index and poorly absorbed ones have a low GI index. The high GI foods are useful to take as recovery after exercise when carbohydrate stores need to be re-stocked quickly, and low GI foods, which have

Table 3.1 High and low GI foods		
	High GI	**Low GI**
Breads	Bagel, wholemeal	Granary, rye bread
Cereals	Bran flakes, Weetabix	Muesli, All-bran
Starches	Baked/mashed potato	Pasta, lentils
Fruit	Watermelon	Apple, peach, pear
Snacks	Jelly beans, rice cakes	Sultanas, Mars bar
Drinks	Sports drinks (isotonic)	Apple/Orange juice

higher fibre contents, release their energy sources more slowly. Examples of high and low GI foods are shown in Table 3.1.

Timing of carbohydrate intake

The timing of when you take the carbohydrate also plays a role in its absorption. Athletes need to experiment with this and it is important to remember that the total carbohydrate intake is the most essential factor.[4]

Before training – take a large meal of high carbohydrate content 2–4 h before training, topped up by a high GI carbohydrate load 30–60 min before. Some athletes do experience gastrointestinal upset with some high GI loads, so do experiment with these, e.g. chicken in pasta with jelly babies, 30 min before training.

During training of more than 1 h duration – take 600–1000 mL of a moderately high GI sports drink that provides fluid as well as carbohydrate loading.

After training – there is a 1–2 h 'window of opportunity' after intensive training when the muscles are particularly receptive to replenishing their stores of glycogen. It is useful to use this time to take in high GI foods to maximise muscle re-fuelling. This is especially important if there is a short gap between training sessions.

'Hitting the wall'

This term is often used in endurance events when, for no apparent reason, the athlete slows down, loses coordination and balance, becomes lightheaded and fatigued and has poor concentration. It may be due to some form of dehydration but it is thought to be due to a sudden depletion of carbohydrate stores and the athlete is therefore 'running on empty'. In endurance training, the body adapts by getting its energy from fat sources rather than carbohydrate sources, thereby conserving the glycogen for the later parts of the race. If there has been inadequate training or the muscle stores of carbohydrate are inadequate at the start of the race due to poor dietary intake during the preceding weeks, then the athlete becomes glycogen depleted and 'hits the wall'.

On a more gradual scale, fatigue can set in over a gradual period of weeks if carbohydrate stores are not replenished after each training session. If the athlete fails to re-stock regularly with high GI foods, then the muscles progressively become depleted of glycogen. If the athlete continues to build up on the training load but ignores his diet, then there comes a point at which there is minimal reserve in the muscles known as 'residual fatigue' and the performance falls and fatigue results. The athlete tries to correct this by intensifying the training, thinking it is a fitness problem but the fatigue worsens and eventually the athlete has to stop training. Being aware of this and spending time re-fuelling after training pays dividends. If residual fatigue has been reached, then the athlete needs to take 2 weeks out from training to rest and re-stock his energy stores with a good carbohydrate and protein diet.

Take home points

- Carbohydrate is the most important energy source.
- Replenishing stores after training is essential.
- Types of carbohydrate and timing of ingestion are crucial.

Proteins

Proteins are needed for the body to repair and rebuild tissues. During activity they are needed for strength, speed and endurance as well as when activity is intensified. However, more is not necessarily better regarding the quantity of protein. Evidence suggests that eating extra protein does not produce more muscle, in fact it is more effective to increase the diet generally (which includes protein and other ingredients) as you intensify the exercise regime rather than increase the protein intake in isolation. Most of us consume enough of the protein we need in our normal diet. Animal sources of protein are richer than non-animal sources and this can be a problem for vegetarian strength and endurance athletes who may need to supplement their protein intake specifically.

Protein supplementation

There are however, a few points to be aware of:

Exercise recovery – as with carbohydrates, there is also a window of opportunity after exercise when the muscles are receptive to absorbing protein. This is a longer window than for carbohydrates but it makes sense to load carbohydrates with proteins after exercise as together they enhance each other's re-fuelling. A protein drink in combination with a rehydration drink after exercise can fulfill this protein need.

Muscle breakdown – if the level of muscle carbohydrate is low, then the muscles will use protein as an energy source resulting in muscle wasting. This may happen even if the protein content in the diet is good. It is important, therefore, to maintain a good carbohydrate intake to 'protect' the muscle mass and protein level.

Take home points

- Most diets have adequate protein contents and supplementation is rarely required.
- Make sure a good overall diet is in place rather than relying on just a lot of protein.
- Timing of protein is also important in refuelling regimes.

FLUIDS

Fluid balance control is as equally important as dietary manipulation in aiding athletes in their quest for better performance. As we exercise, our muscles heat up and sweating via water evaporation is an important method of losing heat. With sweating we lose water and salt (sodium) from the body and during intensive exercise, we should aim to lose only 1–2% of body weight of fluid. Anything greater than that results in dehydration, reduced performance and heat stroke. Therefore, replacing this fluid, either before, during or after exercise is essential. However, this message has been so over-emphasised that, in endurance events, we are witnessing collapse after the races not from dehydration but from over-hydration, which has resulted in dilution of the sodium levels in the blood (aggravated by a high sodium loss in the sweat). So fluids and salt balance is vital for optimum performance.

Generally speaking, we need 2–3 litres (L) of fluids a day.[5] We get 50% from the fluids within our food and 50% directly from fluids drunk. As we exercise we sweat more but as we get fitter we sweat less as we become more efficient at keeping the body cool. We sweat more in hot humid environments and we vary in the degree to which we sweat – there are heavy sweaters, light sweaters, high-salt sweaters and low-salt sweaters – if you taste your sweat and it is very salty you are likely to be a high-salt sweater. Whatever type you are, you need to replace the lost fluid and, as with other dietary ingredients, it is better to start with an adequate level rather than permanently be on 'catch-up'. Likewise, do not rely on your thirst mechanism. This is a poor regulator of fluid balance; unlike many other animals, if we were to rely on our feeling of thirst then we would only replace about 50% of our fluid loss. Once we moisten our mouth then the reflex to drink starts to subside. Generally speaking, a feeling of thirst is a sign of dehydration and you are already playing 'catch up'.

How much is enough fluid?

One of the simplest ways is to weigh yourself before and after training (but before passing urine). A weight loss of 1 kg equates to a 1.2 L loss of fluid. The plan is not to gain weight with too much fluid intake during training. If you cannot weigh yourself, then another method is to observe the colour of your urine throughout the day – this should remain a light yellow colour and not turn dark yellow at any stage, which would mean you are relatively dehydrated.

Planning your drinking

It is important to experiment with your drinking schedule. As most of us know, it is difficult to force several litres of fluid down over a short period of time. Many athletes avoid drinking as they say the resultant passing of urine frequently either upsets their training programme or disturbs their night's sleep. However, we can train our bladder easily if we are patient. If you are taking inadequate fluid intake then plan to increase this over a 7-day period. Initially the bladder will empty more frequently but after a few days it will adapt and expand (it is just a muscle bag after all) and you will find that you revert back to your normal frequency but just pass larger volumes instead. Experiment with timing and types of fluids – which fluids and drinks do you like the taste of best – stick to those as you are more likely to drink the fluids you like. Hydrate yourself early and top up frequently rather than permanently be on 'catch-up'.

A simple fluid regime is as follows:

1. Before exercise
   - Start well hydrated and drink 500 mL sports drink in the 2 hours before exercise
   - Before long endurance events drink 250 mL 15 min before the race starts.
2. During exercise
   - Drink to limit excess sweating; aim for 1–2% weight loss only
   - For exercise over 60 min, aim for 200 mL fluids replacement every 15 min but smaller volumes cause less stomach bloating
   - Work out your strategy before the race based on previous experience; on average a marathon runner will need 2–4 L throughout the race.
3. After exercise
   - Check your weight and drink appropriately
   - Check you have not gained weight with over-hydration
   - Hyponatraemia (too low salt due to over-hydration) can result in nausea, headache, confusion poor coordination and fatigue, which mimics 'hitting the wall' and can delay diagnosis. Prevention and education are better than cure.

What type of drink?

With low to moderate exercise, water or squash is adequate.

During exercise of more than 1 hour a fluid with added carbohydrate such as a sports drink has the added value of reducing fatigue from low energy levels.

After exercise, aim again for a sports drink to replace the fluid and carbohydrates as well as the salt loss in sweating.

Remember, alcohol is not an adequate fluid replacement – it acts as a diuretic giving you the false impression that because you are passing urine you are therefore well hydrated.

Take home points

- Never work on 'catch-up'; start well hydrated and calculate how much you need to rehydrate.
- Plan your rehydration programme from experience not from a book.
- Choose a drink you like that fulfills your needs and stick to it.

THE OTHERS

Minerals and vitamins

There is a massive market and tremendous peer pressure for athletes to feel that taking an extra vitamin or supplementary compound will give them the added extra that will enable them to succeed. There is no real evidence that taking extra minerals and vitamins, on top of a normal healthy diet, will enhance performance and by far the most effective nutritional ingredient in boosting performance is to take a good varied diet. If you exercise intensively you need to increase your diet proportionally as discussed above, and by doing so, you automatically increase the vitamins and minerals you ingest and so there is no need to take extra.

Vitamins

These are divided into fat soluble vitamins (A, D, E, K) which are stored in large amounts in the body. It is very unlikely that anyone will be deficient in these vitamins unless they are on a very restrictive diet or on a totally no-fat diet. There will always be a good store of these vitamins in the body, which is regularly topped-up by a normal diet. Taking extra amounts of these vitamins runs the risk of toxicity and overdose.

Water-soluble vitamins (mainly vitamins B and C groups) are not stored in the body in large amounts and so one could become deficient if, again, one was on a restrictive diet or a diet lacking variety. However, taking more of these vitamins does not boost their effect. Being water soluble, once the limited stores are full, then any excess vitamins are passed out in the urine. So supplementing yourself with vitamins could be interpreted as literally throwing your money down the toilet!

Minerals

These include sodium, potassium, calcium, phosphorus, iron, zinc, magnesium and other lesser minerals. Although they are essential for bodily functions, they are only required in small amounts and, again, a healthy varied diet will easily provide this requirement. More is not necessarily better.

Take home points

- If you stick to a varied healthy diet there is no need to supplement with minerals and vitamins.
- Aim for 4–5 portions of fruit or vegetables a day.

GOING THE EXTRA MILE

- Does taking dietary supplementation enhance performance?
- What is allowed?
- What is safe?
- What are the truths and myths?

Nutritional supplementation has been going on for years, often with little evidence but just in the hope that 'more is better'. It was felt that the same ethos applied to training until over-training syndrome was 'discovered' and now training is tailored to specific activities. So why are so many athletes taking supplements? Look at the facts:

There is widespread use of supplementation – at least 50% of athletes take something 'extra'.

There is massive peer pressure and marketing pressure to take supplements, not just in the sporting world, but in the general public – just go into your local chemist and look at the shelves of vitamins and other ingredients that we now apparently need to function.

Athletes feel that if an opponent is taking something then there is a fear that if you do not take it as well you may be less well equipped to compete. There is very little evidence, however, that supplementation on a broad scale has any performance-enhancing benefit.

Targeted supplementation may have some limited benefit, however, this will only occur if it is on top of a well-balanced diet and fluid intake. Your performance will be very much impaired on the basis of poor carbohydrate, protein, fat and fluids intake, rather than whether you have not taken your added supplements that day.

Diet supplementation is not a compromise for a poor diet and you would do better to improve the diet rather than take more supplements.

More is not better – be aware of the risks of toxicity.

Be aware also that supplements are not governed by the same strict quality controlled systems that pharmaceutical companies go through to produce a medicine. Many supplements, as much as 40% in some studies, are contaminated with other ingredients not listed on the bottle, many of which will be on the World Anti-Doping Agency (WADA) banned listings.[6] So you may be taking a banned substance without knowing it.

TARGETED SUPPLEMENTATION

Energy

We have already discussed the role of carbohydrate loading and re-fuelling. This is a form of dietary supplementation that has been proven to enhance performance by topping up and re-stocking the glycogen muscle stores.

Creatine

This exists as part of the ATP-CP instant energy source for short quick explosive activity. Creatine comes from meat and fish and enhances muscle mass and improves recovery between repeated bouts of high intensity exercise. Supplementing more than you get from a normal diet has been shown to improve performance but with prolonged use, there is still concern over the effect on the kidneys. If you are involved in explosive sports with short bouts of high intensity, then a loading course of 4–5 days followed by a maintenance dose for 3 months maximum at a selected part of your training season, has been shown to be beneficial.

Bicarbonate

Theoretically this acts as an alkaline to neutralise the lactic acid that builds up in anaerobic metabolism and causes muscle fatigue. Studies have shown it to be beneficial, but only in the short term and the effect is negated by the gastrointestinal side-effects of the bicarbonate which often make it unpalatable. Some studies have shown sodium citrate to have similar effects.

Caffeine

Studies have shown caffeine to enhance the performance in short-term high intensity exercise as well as in the later stages of prolonged exercise by acting as a stimulant on the nervous system and also enhancing mobilisation of fat for energy. It is present in coffee and tea but also many common beverages. Its side-effects include headaches, racing heart rates, insomnia, shaking and tremor and stomach upsets. It is not banned by WADA but is monitored at present so that WADA can see if it is being increasingly used and possibly abused by athletes.

Immune protection

Moderate exercise regimes on a regular basis have been shown to enhance the body's immune system, however, prolonged and heavy exercise regimes can depress the immune response to infection. This effect is enhanced if you are on a poor diet. Many supplements have been advocated to correct this and 'protect' the athletes throughout intensive training, such as antioxidants. Glutamine, zinc, Echinacea, probiotics and colostrums have been used in the past, however, there is no real evidence to support this approach. A good diet would be more worthwhile.

Glucosamine and chondroitin

Claims that this combination acts to repair cartilage, supplement the synovial fluid and reduce the pain and swelling of osteoarthritic joints are not confirmed in studies on either side of the Atlantic. There is no evidence that these supplements act as a protective measure. However, there is no doubt that a lot of athletes, both young and old, find benefit from taking these and some studies have shown improved mobility and function in osteoarthritic joints.

Take home points

- A good healthy varied diet is the key – there are no quick fixes with supplementation.
- Studies show that most supplements are ineffective.
- Be aware of the toxic effects of some supplements and that many are contaminated with other substances that may have doping risks.

MAXIMISING PERFORMANCE

Having discussed the theory of nutritional advice, how do we put this into action? The key to improving performance through diet is to have good planning. Plan and prepare the pre-match intake, what you are going to take on board during the event and how you are going to re-fuel afterwards. All the planning should be done well in advance. There is no benefit to leaving things to the last minute or experimenting on the day of competition. You need to know what foods and drinks you need and which ones you like and have them ready to take at the correct times.

Pre-exercise

We have discussed the merits of maximising the carbohydrate stores in the muscles and the liver on a regular basis as part of your training programme, not only as a baseline ingredient, but also during the window of opportunity after training to re-stock the stores. This prevents residual fatigue and starts you off on a firm base (Fig. 3.8).

Building up to competition you need to enhance the stores by 'carbo-loading' for 2–3 days before the event, especially if the event lasts more than 1 hour.[7] As you reduce the training load, you increase the carbohydrate intake. See Box 3.1 for the types of food you need to include for this.

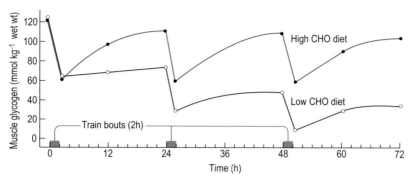

Figure 3.8 The influences of dietary carbohydrates on muscle glycogen stores during repeated days of training.

Box 3.1 **Types of food for carbo-loading**

Breakfast
- Cereal with semi-skimmed milk
- Bread/pancakes with jam or honey
- Fruit juice

Snack
- Jaffa cakes or muffins
- Fruit
- Fluids – isotonic
- Jelly beans/sugary sweets

Lunch
- Bread, pizza or baked potato
- Fruit and yoghurt

Snack
- Pancake with jam
- Fruit
- Sports drink

Evening meal
- Pasta with chicken
- Fruit
- Ice cream
- Fluids

Pre-match meal

Three hours before the event, eat a high carbohydrate meal to stock up stores and replace any lost overnight. Work out what suits you best both in terms of taste and timing. Some athletes have a fast digestive transit and others are slow – the latter may cause stomach cramps if the timing is not right for you. If the event is early in the morning you will not have time to have a meal 3 hours before, so snacks of high carbohydrate supplemented with sports drinks may be required instead. Examples of pre-match meals:

4 slices of bread with jam or honey and a sports drink

or

plate of pasta and tomato sauce

or

bowl of cereal with sultanas and bananas

or

baked potato with baked beans.

During exercise

Aim to top up with 300–500 mL of a sports drink 15 min before a 1 hour event. Work out which you prefer to 'sample' frequently during an event – either water or sports drink – the sports drink has the added advantage of carbohydrate and sodium but is not palatable for some. High GI foods/snacks are also preferable.

Recovery

As discussed previously, make use of this 'window of opportunity' to re-fuel on fluids, then carbohydrate and protein sources within 1–2 hours of exercise.

Take home points

- Plan your nutritional programme – do not leave it to the last moment.
- Maximise your stores before the day of the event.
- Do not forget the fluids.

CLINICAL CASE

A 47-year-old-female Cypriot amateur marathon runner comes into your clinic asking for advice. She is an experienced marathon runner having run eight previous marathons in both New York and London in a time of just under 4 hours. She is training for the London marathon which is 4 weeks away now but her training has been hampered by work commitments which have taken her abroad recently. She has followed her usual training regime for the last 4 months otherwise. This year she plans to run with her 18-year-old son who is a good athlete but who has been unwell with a persistent sore throat.

Everything had been going well with her training up until 10 days ago when, as she started to increase her speed sessions, she has noticed herself becoming fatigued and lacking energy. Her times have fallen and she has felt worse as she has tried to intensify her training. She says she eats well but is disinterested in food, her sleep pattern is poor but she puts that down to pressures at work. Her weight is stable and there are no fevers but the occasional night sweats. She has not had any periods for 18 months but her sister stopped her periods at the age of 44. She has no other systemic symptoms but does admit she is despondent and anxious about her symptoms and her ability to be able to run in the marathon and does not want to let her son down. She is on no regular drugs or supplements and has no relevant past medical history.

Examination is basically normal. She is a slim woman who is slightly pale but who has no lymph node enlargement in neck, axillae or abdomen. There are no other positive physical findings.

- What other questions do you want to ask her?
- What is your differential diagnosis?
- Are there any tests you would want to perform?
- How would you manage this woman?

There are many reasons why this woman may be fatigued and it is the role of the physician to explore these options in both the history and examination with a view to giving pointers for further investigation.

In no particular order, her diagnosis could be related to the following causes:

Infection – has she picked up a viral infection possibly from her son who may be harbouring a glandular-fever like illness or are there any other sources of infection: low grade enteritis, urinary tract or respiratory?

Over-training – or unexplained underperformance syndrome (UUPS): this is an objective loss of performance without a medical cause despite 2 weeks rest often associated with intensive training in endurance athletes associated with frequent minor infections. Fatigue is the predominant symptom but also there are sweats, bowel habit changes, elevated heart rate and insomnia. There are no blood tests to confirm the diagnosis although elevated cortisol levels and neutrophil levels give a suggestion. Diagnosis is often after excluding other causes and treatment is via a multidisciplinary approach through diet and retraining.

Diet – as we have outlined in this chapter, diet plays a major role in performance, in the type, quantity, timing and re-fuelling of energy stores. It is important to enquire in great detail about every aspect of your patient's dietary intake, so as to reassure yourself there is no nutritional cause.

Depression – do not forget about issues that may not have anything to do with the patient's sporting aspirations. Depression could lead to all this woman's symptoms, be it in reaction to a physical, psychological, social, financial or work orientated issues.

Drugs – although this woman is not on any medication, do not forget that medication can cause fatigue symptoms, e.g. beta blockers for hypertension.

Systemic conditions – below is a list of systemic conditions that may cause fatigue and need to be excluded, some of which may not be relevant in this case:

- Hypothyroidism
- Cardiac conditions – arrhythmias, HOCM
- Anaemia of a variety of causes including thalassaemias
- Diabetes
- Hepatitis
- Colitis/coeliac disease
- Hormonal – moving into a menopausal state can cause fatigue and night sweats.

In this woman, blood tests including FBP, ESR, glandular fever and Coxsackie virus screens, U&E, LFT, TFT, calcium, fasting cortisol, FSH, LH and oestradiol, iron studies and thalassaemia and coeliac screens were all normal. After further discussion, it became apparent that she had not been re-fuelling after her training sessions and over a 4-week period, her life had become so busy she had not paid attention to her carbohydrate intake. The blood results were reassuring for her and after some nutritional education and time spent to replenish glycogen stores, she made a quick recovery and managed to complete the marathon in a good time together with her son.

REFERENCES

1. Burke LM, Kiens B, Ivy JL. Carbohydrates and fat for training and recovery. J Sports Sci 2004; 22(1):15–30.
2. Stear SJ. Fuelling fitness for sports performance: sports nutrition guide. London: Sugar Bureau; 2004.
3. Foster H. Easy GI diet: use the glycaemic index to lose weight and gain energy. London: Hamlyn; 2004.
4. Williams C, Serratosa L. Nutrition on match day [soccer players]. J Sports Sci 2006; 24(7):687–697.
5. Buskirk ER, Phul SM. Body fluid balance: exercise and sport. London: CRC Press; 1996.
6. WADA regulations. Online. Available: www.didglobal.com.
7. Bussau VA, Fairchild TJ, Rao A et al. Carbohydrate loading in human muscle: an improved 1 day protocol. Eur J Appl Physiol 2002; 87(3):290–295.

Chapter | 4 |

Drugs and sport

© 2009 Elsevier Ltd, Inc, BV
DOI: 10.1016/B978-0-443-06813-3.00007-7

INTRODUCTION

The use of drugs to enhance sporting performance, and the fight by the authorities to try and detect those athletes seen as cheating by using performance-enhancing drugs, is a major problem within sport today. This is not just confined to professional sport but has consequences throughout the world of sport, both recreational and amateur, in that professional athletes often pave the way and set an example for recreational athletes. Despite increasing investment and technology aimed to detect drug abuse within the sport, the taking of drugs within professional sport is widespread[1] and unfortunately, the authorities always seem to be one step behind the athletes.

The International Olympic Committee (IOC)[2] defines drug doping as 'the use of a substance or method which is potentially harmful to an athlete's health, or is capable of enhancing their performance, or the presence in the athlete's body of a prohibited substance, or evidence of the use thereof, or evidence of the use of a prohibited method'.

It is interesting to point out that in the IOC's definition, the first and most important aspect is to protect the athlete from the harmful effects of drugs. Obviously it is important to prevent the cheats from gaining improved performance; however, the overriding issue is to protect the athletes from being harmed by potentially dangerous drugs, when their insight into these effects may be clouded by the goal to achieve better performances.

Historically, performance-enhancing drugs date back many years, even to ancient times when Greeks, Romans and Egyptians used potions and herbal mixtures to try and improve performance. Doping was evidenced in the nineteenth century when stimulants were used, both for athletes and for military troops to help performance. A series of cyclists tragically died in both the Olympic events and the Tour de France, most notably Kurt Yensen in 1960 and Tommy Simpson in 1967. The IOC set up a medical commission in 1967 and started drug testing in the 1968 Mexico Olympics.

Anabolic steroids in the form of testosterone can be dated back to the 1920s and again were used in the Second World War by German troops, to enhance their aggressive nature. In the world of sport it was first alleged to be used in the 1950s in power events, such as lifting, throwing and wrestling. In the 1970s the IOC started testing for anabolic steroids. The most notable athlete who was found positive for this was Ben Johnson in the 1988 Seoul Olympics. In the late 1980s the set-up of the Australian Sports Drug Agency spread the net from in-competition testing to out-of-competition testing and random drug testing on athletes. At the same time, it became apparent that athletes were using other forms of doping, such as re-infusing blood and later in the 1990s, using erythropoietin (EPO) to enhance oxygen carrying capacity. Blood doping was banned by the IOC in 1986; in the Sydney Olympics EPO was detected for the first time.

In 1999, the World Anti-Doping Agency (WADA)[3] was established under the initiative of the IOC and now represents the world authority and regulatory body on drug doping. On 1 January every year, it issues a complete list of prohibited drugs, with alterations from the previous year. It is important for the athlete as well as the team physician and sports physician to be familiar with any alterations that occur to this list.

So why do we test for drug doping?

This is done for three main reasons: first, to deter athletes from being tempted to take drugs that can not only cause the side-effects, but can have a serious implication on their short and long-term health. Second, it is performed to deter any cheating. The ethos of competitive sport is that it is performed on a baseline of equal opportunity and training benefit, rather than the ability to take drugs to enhance performance. Third, it performs as a reminder to athletes of the doping regulations, to ensure they avoid the inadvertent use of banned drugs.

Why do athletes take drugs?

With the knowledge that WADA is out there to detect medication abuse, and that there is both in- and out-of-competition testing that can occur at any time, and that it can be harmful to your health, why do athletes take the risk of taking performance-enhancing drugs? There is little evidence behind the reasons for this; however the following reasons may represent the multifactorial issues involved.

1. To succeed at all costs. For a professional athlete, the opportunity of reaching their goal and achieving greatness in their sporting activity, can override any other issue within their life, both short and long term. A survey was performed, just on Olympic athletes, in which the athletes were asked if they would take a banned but undetectable performance-enhancing drug that would ensure their success in competitions over the next 5 years, if they were offered the drug. Despite being fully informed of its dangers including its eventually leading to premature death, 60% said they would have no hesitation in taking the drug.[4] This highlights the short-term goals that these athletes have to the detriment of any long-term consequences. One could call this a higher level of focus, but this may give some insight into why some athletes take banned medication to achieve their goals.
2. The knowledge that other athletes or their competitors are also taking medication. At the top level of sport the difference between winning and losing is so fine, that if you think or believe that your competitors are taking any form of ergogenic drugs, that you will have less chance of winning.
3. Expectation from others. There may be pressure from peers, coaches or parents to take medication to produce 'your best performance', so as to not let anybody else down.
4. Financial rewards and security. If taking medications means you win your goal and therefore receive financial rewards and security for your family and future, then there may be increased pressure to take these medications.
5. Lack of knowledge and education. This should not be an issue due to the increased awareness that athletes have and the access via the internet and other agencies to ask advice on medication, however, in some countries where access to legal and medication advice may be limited, ignorance may be a cause, although not a genuine reason.

It is likely that a combination of the above explains why athletes take banned medications. Ignorance, however, is no excuse, either from the athlete or his advising physician. However, the athlete needs to be made aware that at the end of the day it is he, and he alone, that is responsible for ingesting or taking any medication that may be banned. Likewise it is he, and he alone, who has to explain how medication got into his body, and it is he, and he alone, that will suffer the resulting consequences.

Getting access to banned drugs is not difficult from either the internet or from colleagues. The ingestion of anabolic steroids among bodybuilders is not uncommon,[5] often as a result of dissatisfaction with body image in a similar way that anorexia can affect young females. The attraction of increased muscle tone and power to offset personality deficiencies can be attractive and the 'stacking' of medication, when two drugs are given together via different routes, either orally or intramuscularly, or the 'shot-gunning' of drugs when several preparations are taken at once, is practised. The practice of 'short-gauge', when injecting an individual muscle is performed to enhance that particular muscle definition, can result in ruptures of the collagen fibres and tendon tearing. Unfortunately, 'plateauing' occurs when there is failure to get further gain from taking medication, and the temptation then is to increase the dose, which unfortunately only results in further side-effects. As a result of this, 'cycling' is performed and drugs are taken for anything from 4–18 months with a 2–3 month rest period. Unfortunately, dependence, be it physical or psychological, can occur. It is important to tell athletes that there are no safe anabolic steroids.

PROHIBITED SUBSTANCES

The list of prohibited substances is produced by WADA every year and the reader is encouraged to read this list from the WADA website to at least become familiar with the different types of medications. It is beyond the scope of this book to discuss every form of medication but we will highlight the groups of drugs, their perceived effects, their side-effects and some common medications within this group to illustrate the size of the problem. It is important for each team physician, and the athletes themselves, to be 100% sure that every form of medication that they prescribe or take is not on the banned list. This is especially important for over-the-counter medications and for combinations of drugs that may contain small quantities of banned substances. It is also important to be aware that products that are 'safe' in one country may not be the same 'safe' products in another country. It is important to research all the ingredients of every product to be absolutely sure they are not on the banned list. One useful website for information to clarify whether a product is banned in or out of competition is the website *www.didglobal.com* and athletes should be encouraged to explore this website.

This list of prohibited substances and methods includes four categories, as follows:

A. Prohibited substances in and out of competition
  A1. anabolic agent
  A2. hormones and related substances
  A3. beta 2 agonists
  A4. agents with antioestrogenic activity
  A5. diuretics and other masking agents
B. Prohibited classes of substances in competition only:
  B1. stimulants
  B2. narcotics
  B3. cannabinoids
  B4. glucocorticosteroids

C. Prohibited methods in and out of competition:
   C1. enhancement of oxygen transfer
   C2. chemical and physical manipulations
   C3. gene doping
D. Substances whose ingredients vary tremendously from product to product and within the same product when found overseas; it is therefore very important to read the ingredients of any form of medication and to make sure they are not on the prohibited list. One drug that has recently been removed from the prohibited list is pseudoephedrine, otherwise known in the UK as Sudafed which is a commonly found cough and cold decongestant. There have been many cases of athletes inadvertently taking this medication as part of a cough and cold cure, and in the last 12 months, this too has been removed from the prohibited list, but has been maintained on the monitoring programme. Excessive levels of pseudoephedrine or caffeine may signify a return of these products back onto the prohibited list.

Prohibited substances in and out of competition

Anabolic agents

Anabolic androgenic steroids occur naturally in the body and are secreted by the testes, ovaries and adrenal glands. They are responsible for the development of secondary sexual characteristics, however, testosterone promotes aggressive behaviour. Anabolic androgenic steroids (AASs) are derivatives of testosterone and many derivatives of testosterone have been used by athletes in the past (e.g. Androlone, stanozolol) and are banned. Athletes have used these drugs for strength events such as powerlifting, wrestling and sprinting and throwing in the track and field arena, but they are used widely and more worryingly, have drifted into the recreational field of sports and are known to be used by teenagers to develop muscle bulk.[6-9]

The drugs (or 'gear') are taken orally or intramuscularly either in a cyclical manner or taken via the two routes together ('stacking') or in several preparations at once ('shot-gunning'). Occasionally a person may 'short-gauge' by injecting an individual muscle group specifically, as seen in bodybuilders. Most AASs are available on the internet or via gyms but there is a real problem in education of both professional and recreational athletes as to their short- and long-term effects.

The methods by which AASs affect the body are as follows:

Anabolic effect. This induces protein synthesis in skeletal muscles, thus increasing muscle bulk and strength.
Anti-catabolic effect. In a period of intensive training when improvements in training are limited by the catabolic effect of glucocorticosteroids, this effect is minimised by AASs and permits increased training load.
Encouraging aggression. By increasing aggression and competitive nature, this encourages greater training intensity and better performance both in and out of competition.

Side-effects

The side-effects of anabolic steroids are extremely common. Most are reversible on cessation of the drug, however, some significant and some serious side-effects have been reported and some deaths are known. In one study, mortality among powerlifts because of steroid abuse was significantly higher than in a control population; 12.9% versus 3.1% and in another study, steroid use was shown to result in increased risk from violent death with impulsive, aggressive or depressive behaviour. This is often known as 'roid rage'. There is also the risk of sharing infection if the drugs are administered intramuscularly and needles are shared. The risk of HIV, hepatitis and deep muscular abscess formation is well known among needle-sharers. The side-effects within both sexes include acne, alopecia, hypertension, irritability, mood swings with aggression and changes in libido. Among men, there is a reduced sperm count and reduction in testicular size as well as marked gynaecomastia. In women, there is hirsutism, menstrual irregularities, male pattern baldness and deepening of the voice, and in adolescents, there is increased body and facial hair, acne and premature closure of the epiphysis, resulting in stunted growth.

More specifically within the liver, in both sexes, abuse of anabolic steroids can cause liver disorders, including raised liver enzymes and hyperbilirubinaemia with biliary obstruction and jaundice, which can take up to 3 months to reverse. Similarly, the use of anabolic steroids can affect the cholesterol balance by raising the LDL and lowering the HDL/LDL ratio which is a risk factor towards heart disease and myocardial infarction.

Interestingly, cases of tumour formation in athletes using anabolic steroids, including Wilms tumour, prostate cancer and leukaemia have been reported, although a direct link has not been made. Blood pressure rises have also been associated with AAS intake and this, together with the cholesterol, puts the athlete at risk of coronary thrombosis. As mentioned above, acne formation together with sebaceous cysts and folliculitis is not uncommon among athletes taking anabolic steroids. Care should be taken when prescribing tetracycline or isotretinoin as treatment for these conditions, as these drugs may also aggravate pre-existing liver damage. Many of these side-effects are reversible on cessation of the drugs, however, it is important to educate the athletes of these side-effects and that they are putting themselves at risk of long-term problems.

Hormones and related substances

The following substances are prohibited:

Erythropoietin (EPO), a naturally occurring hormone secreted by the kidney. Its role is to increase red cell production and red cell mass and its use is mainly in patients with anaemia due to chronic disease such as chronic renal failure to enhance oxygen transfer. The effect of EPO in sport is to increase the oxygen carrying capacity which therefore causes an increase in energy production in aerobic oxidation of glucose. This is most important in endurance athletes and that is why it has been abused within cyclists and cross-country skiers. Side-effects of EPO include increasing the MCV of the blood and therefore its viscosity level. This makes blood more likely to congeal and increases the risk of myocardial infarction and cerebrovascular accident. This effect is increased if the athlete is dehydrated. Less commonly, side-effects can include fever, headaches, anxiety and lethargy. Before WADA were able to detect levels of EPO in athletes, the only way of detecting it was to measure the haematocrit level in the blood; however, this was rather unsatisfactory as normal values can vary tremendously. More recently (since the Sydney Olympics) blood and urine samples have been able to identify new exogenous forms of EPO.[10,11]

Human growth hormone (HGH) is a hormone produced by the pituitary gland and is essential for growth and development. It has an anabolic nature and causes an increase in protein synthesis and reduction in protein catabolism, thus improving muscle strength and size. It also decreases the rate of glucose utilisation. HGH stimulates the production of insulin-like growth factor I (IGF-1) in the liver, which together with HGH produces this effect. HGH is species-specific and therefore human HGH can only benefit humans, whereas bovine or porcine HGH has no effect on humans. The use of HGH from cadavers led to the risk of mad cow disease so, more recently, artificial HGH has been used. Athletes use HGH to increase muscle mass and strength although studies to confirm this are very small. Side-effects include acromegaly in adult athletes, hypothyroidism, hypercholesterolaemia, ischaemic heart disease, cardiomyopathy, diabetes, osteoporosis and menstrual disorders.[12]

Insulin-like growth factors (IGF). IGF-1 is used by athletes with the aim of increasing muscle mass. However, studies have been limited and this effect is yet to be proven. Unfortunately, IGF-1 levels have been linked to prostate, rectal and lung cancers because it is thought to be mitogenic.

Human chorionic gonadotropin (HCG). HCG is produced by the placenta and has a similar structure to luteinising hormone which stimulates ovulation in the females, and interstitial cell production and testosterone in males. It is therefore sometimes taken by athletes on the assumption that it can increase testosterone levels; however, this would be detected through a raised testosterone–epitestosterone (T/E) ratio.

Insulin. Insulin is anabolic in nature causing cell growth and increasing glucose amino acid uptake and increasing protein synthesis. It is used among power sport athletes in bodybuilding and weightlifting, often in combination with anabolic steroids. Most abusers inject 10 units of regular insulin after exercise and then consume large amounts of sugar-containing foods and drinks. The effect of hyperinsulinaemic states in athletes is not well supported, however, it is meant to stimulate amino acid transport in human muscle and inhibit protein breakdown, thus increasing body muscle mass. It is difficult to detect, as human insulin only lasts in the body for 10 min and so detection is almost impossible.

Beta 2 agonists

Beta 2 agonists such as salbutamol, terbutaline and salmeterol are used mainly in the aerosol form for treatment of asthma, however, when given by injection they have an anabolic effect and are not allowed by the oral or intravenous route and are therefore prohibited. In excessive doses their side-effects include tremor, tachycardia, palpitations, headache, nausea, vomiting and nervousness. As described below, these drugs can be given in an inhaled form when accompanied by a therapeutic use exemption (TUE) form. However, like most TUE forms if these drugs are found in the system in a concentration that is deemed excessive for normal therapeutic use, then further investigation will be instigated. For example, if an athlete falsely assumes that excessive doses of salbutamol, by inhaled form, will give him anabolic benefit, then he may have excessive levels in his blood system and urine as detected by blood testing.

Agents with antioestrogenic activity

These drugs are used differently by males and females and consist of several different types of medications. Aromatase inhibitors lower the amount of oestrogen within the body, whereas selective oestrogen receptor modulators (SERMS) block the oestrogen receptors; other drugs including toremifene and tamoxifen[13] have antioestrogenic effects.

Male athletes use these drugs mainly to prevent the development of gynaecomastia which develops as a result of the side-effects of anabolic steroids. There is also a small benefit of increasing the testosterone level in males. In females, there is evidence that tamoxifen has a masculinising effect, however, it has also been shown to be harmful and increases the risk of thromboembolism.

Diuretics and other masking agents

Diuretics are used in events where weight limits are set. These include weightlifting, horseracing, judo, wrestling and boxing. Drugs such as diuretics, as well as other dehydration techniques such as exercising in hot conditions, food and water restrictions and sauna exposure, can dehydrate an athlete and keep his weight below a target weight. The risks of these are that there may be rapid dehydration and electrolyte disturbance, which may be harmful to the athlete.

Epitestosterone. Taken by athletes who are also taking testosterone or anabolic steroids in an attempt to increase the epitestosterone level within the body and therefore normalise the testosterone–epitestosterone (T/E) ratio. It has been mentioned that a ratio greater than four will signify excessive exogenous testosterone, so increasing the epitestosterone level will therefore reduce the ratio.

Probenecid is used clinically to increase the excretion of uric acid in patients who suffer from gout. It can also be used to accelerate the excretion of prohibited drugs and, therefore, if found in the body without a TUE form may suggest an attempt to increase excretion of prohibited substances. Finasteride is used clinically in the treatment of prostatic hypertrophy and male pattern baldness. It is also used in athletes who suffer male pattern baldness as a result of excessive testosterone and anabolic steroid use, in an attempt to mask this physical side-effect of the steroids. Plasma volume expanders are used to dilute concentration of haemoglobin seen as a result of taking EPO. EPO increases the amount of haemoglobin and MCV and plasma volume expanders reduce this effect to try and mask the use of EPO.

Prohibited classes of substances in competition only

Stimulants

There is a vast group of stimulants that are included in the WADA prohibited list and, up until recently, all were on the prohibited list. Caffeine, a naturally found component of coffee, was theoretically banned and there was confusion as to what level was acceptable. In 2004, caffeine, phenylephrine and pseudoephedrine were removed from the prohibited list but are still being measured in drug testing and monitored to see if their use is excessive.

Amphetamines

Amphetamines have been used clinically in the treatment of narcolepsy and attention deficit disorders seen in children. They are seen to have a beneficial effect in athletes by reducing fatigue, increasing alertness, aggression, hostility and competitiveness, and apparently it is felt to give an edge in speed and endurance events. Its side-effects include arrhythmias and blood pressure control difficulties, as well as behavioural side-effects including irritability, restlessness, disinterest and tremor. In excessive doses there may be rapid hypertension, angina and also cerebral haemorrhage. There may also be loss of judgement and difficulty in cooling down.

Cocaine

Cocaine is a stimulant very much like amphetamines and carries with it the same side-effect profile of cardiac arrhythmias, myocardial infarction, cerebral haemorrhage and convulsions. Its positive effects on athletic performance are minimal but its biggest problem lies in recreational use among society. In many countries, it is illegal both to use and possess cocaine; WADA in support of this have put it on the banned list.

Modafinil

Up until recently this was not on WADA's prohibited list but has been added, as it was discovered athletes were using it. It is, however, used clinically in the treatment of narcolepsy and if a patient of yours has this condition, and is taking this medication then they should apply for a TUE which requires the diagnosis of narcolepsy to be confirmed by a specialist after confirmation by sleep studies.

Narcotics

Narcotics are used clinically in the management of moderate to severe pain, and include morphine, pethidine and diamorphine. They have no ergogenic effect but, as pain killers, can mask pain and allow athletes to compete while injured. It is for this reason that they are on the prohibited list. Other related forms of medications, including codeine, dextromethorphan, dihydrocodeine, Vicodin and tramadol, are permitted.

Cannabinoids

Cannabinoids such as marijuana, cannabis and hash are prohibited in competitions. Cannabis is a commonly used recreational drug, but not many athletes realise that in chronic users, it can stay in the body for a prolonged period of time. In occasional users, metabolites of cannabis can be detected in the urine 5–7 days after exposure, however, in chronic users it may be detected for as long as 30 days after the last exposure. This is important for the athlete to be aware of because he could have taken the substance several weeks before a competition, only to be tested positive in the competition weeks later.

There are no performance-enhancing effects of cannabis, however, it may have a calming effect in some people. Cannabis is rapidly absorbed through the lungs and in view of this fact there is a risk that passive smokers of cannabis may inadvertently have a positive drug test. For this reason, cannabis has been included in the list of drugs subject to certain restrictions and a concentration level up to 15 ng/mL of carboxy-tetrahydrocannabinol has been allowed to account for this fact.

Glucocorticosteroids

All glucocorticosteroids are prohibited in competition when administered orally, rectally or by intravenous or intramuscular injection. If their use is, however, clinically required, this has to be accompanied by a standard TUE form. Topical use of corticosteroids, whether it be nasal, via the skin, buccal, or via the eye, ear or mouth are not prohibited and do not require any form of TUE. Inhaled corticosteroids require an on-line declaration via the 100% ME website (*www.100percentme. co.uk*). The ergogenic effect of glucocorticosteroids is limited. There is some speculation that they may cause muscle hypertrophy and increased cardiac output, however, the evidence is limited. The side-effect profile, however, is far greater with harmful effects on the blood pressure, sugar balance and vascular system, including variable effects on mood. Because glucocorticosteroids are used in a variety of antiinflammatory conditions, the physician needs to be fully aware of which drugs, via which form, are allowed, whether they be accompanied by a standard TUE form or an on-line declaration.

Prohibited methods in and out of competition

Enhancement of oxygen transfer

This includes blood doping and artificial oxygen carriers.

Blood doping is the administration of blood or red blood cells to an athlete to increase the red blood cell mass. This can be autologous when the athlete's own blood is transfused back into himself or homogenous when appropriately donated blood is used. This method was used prior to the development of EPO as a form of increasing the oxygen carrying capacity of the blood. 2–3 units of the athlete's own blood is removed 6 weeks prior to competition and then re-infused a day or two before competition, thus bolstering the red cell mass. The risks of blood doping include allergic reactions to donor blood and the method is detected via raised red cell mass and haematocrit value within the blood test.

One recent issue that has become apparent with this form of blood doping has been the therapeutic use of autologous blood injection when treating forms of tendinopathy. A recent form of treatment in chronic tendinopathy is to inject, under ultrasound control 1–2 mL of the patient's own blood into the area of hypoechogenicity within the tendon. This has been performed with either spun or unspun blood products. This is blood doping and according to WADA is prohibited; however, it has been increasingly used as a form of treatment of chronic tendinopathy and may be discussed by WADA in their annual review.

Artificial oxygen carriers. These blood substitutes are used clinically in the management of hypovolaemic shock and prevention of ischaemic tissue damage. They are used in emergency situations where cross-matching of blood is unavailable or time consuming. The contents of these products are biochemically modified haemoglobin molecules which, in theory, are meant to increase oxygen uptake. Their use among sports athletes is unknown and their effect is also unknown.

Chemical or physical manipulation

This group includes any tampering of the urine sampling process such as sample substitution using surrogate urine, or the use of previous past urine samples from the athlete. Similarly, intravenous infusions in an attempt to dilute blood levels are also prohibited except in acute medical emergencies.

Gene doping

The use of gene doping or gene transfer to improve performance is a potential concern for WADA and there have been two meetings sponsored by WADA, in March 2002 in New York and December 2005 in Stockholm. The threat is real, although in its infancy, but enough to say that any athlete or physician involved in gene transfer procedures with athletes is banned.

Classes of drugs banned in certain sports

Alcohol

Alcohol is not a performance-enhancing drug and has a negative effect on performance by impairing reaction time, hand/eye coordination and gross motor skills. It is, however, prohibited in competition only in certain sports. These include power boating, motorcycling, modern pentathlon (involving shooting), karate, pool, billiards, aeronautics, archery and automobiles. The reason behind this is that impairing coordination may have a dangerous effect on the participants and spectators.

Beta blockers

Beta blockers are prohibited only in the following sports: aeronautics, archery (also out of competition), automobile, billiards, pool, bridge, chess, gymnastics, modern pentathlon (involving shooting), motorcycling, 9-pin bowling, sailing (match race rounds only), shooting, skiing, snowboarding and wrestling.

Beta blockers are used clinically for the management of hypertension, arrhythmias, migraine, anxiety and tremor. Their anxiolytic and anti-tremor effects can be seen as beneficial in sports such as shooting and archery, and where a steady hand is needed. Apart from this they do not have a performance-enhancing effect.

DRUG TESTING PROCEDURE

The drug testing process is ultimately controlled by WADA but this is commonly outsourced to other agencies such as UK sport. It is important for the sports physician dealing with the athlete or the team to be familiar with the process and regulations of drug testing, as any alteration in the procedure or deviation from the regulations may put an athlete at risk or invalidate the testing process. Increasingly nowadays, athletes are required to inform the doping regulators of their whereabouts both in and out of competition so that testing can occur randomly. Increasingly, tests are not being performed out of competition.

Selection process

An athlete can be selected at any time to be subject to a testing process. This may be because they have been targeted by the doping authorities or chosen at random out of competition. During competition, for example in team sports, the doping agency should arrive 1 hour before kick off/start and, together with representatives from both teams, make a random selection of players from both teams to be tested at the end of the competition. The selection process is anonymous so that representatives are unaware of which players they are selecting, and representatives are not informed as to which players are due to be tested.

Notification

An athlete can be notified of their selection for drug testing either in person, in or out or competition, or by telephone or written notice when out of competition. If notified during competition the drug tester will identify himself to the athlete and record the athlete's details on a notification form, which is then signed by the athlete. A copy is then kept by both parties and signifies to the athlete that he acknowledges that he has been accepted for drug testing and will comply with the testing process. A refusal to sign this form or to present for drug testing will be regarded as a positive test and the athlete will be subjected to penalisation. Once the athlete has been notified he does not need to go immediately to the drug testing station but, in the presence of a chaperone may cool-down, compete in further events if required and if appropriate, fulfil media commitments, attend a victory ceremony, or if necessary receive medical attention. During this time, he can eat and drink, and sealed drinks are provided by the drug testers for them to rehydrate themselves.

Sample collection

Once the athlete feels he is prepared to give a sample, then he attends the drug control station. This whole process and the sealing of the sample should be performed solely by the athlete with no interference other than instruction from the drug testing official. The bottles provided should be appropriately sealed and numbered and the facilities available should be uniform throughout. The athlete's representative, usually the team physician, is permitted to observe the whole process, except the actual collection of the sample. However, the sample collection has to be witnessed by the drug control official who should be the same gender as the athlete. Having chosen a suitable sealed urine sample receptacle, the athlete produces a minimum of 100 mL of urine. If there is insufficient sample, the initial sample is sealed with a temporary seal and additional samples collected and mixed with the original sample. The athlete is required to wear gloves so as to prevent the adding of masking agents from beneath the fingernails. Following collection of the sample, the athlete returns to the doping control station where he will be taken through the process by the doping control official, together with a second official as witness, and the athlete's representative. The athlete will be asked to select a sample testing kit which consists of two bottles labelled A and B. It is important to check that the kits are sealed correctly and that the bottles have not been used, and that they have suitable untamperable lids. The urine is poured into bottles A and B leaving a small amount in the sample bottle. The athlete himself seals the bottles with self-sealing lids and confirms that all the bottle numbers correspond to what is written on the form. During this process, the drug testing official will document volumes and timing of samples. The drug testing official will also check the pH and specific gravity of the sample using a multistick testing strip. If the urine is more acidic than 5.0 or more alkaline than 9.0 or has a specific gravity of less than 1.010, a second sample is required. Once the samples have been provided and the bottles sealed back in the polystyrene case, the athlete is asked to provide a medical declaration to list all the medications taken over the previous week, be they over-the-counter medications, prescribed drugs or any other forms of medication including vitamins and supplements, and whether they were administered in any form whether by mouth, injection, inhalation, suppository, nasal spray or topical application. It is vitally important to list all the drugs taken and if there is any doubt, to specify the circumstances on this part of the form. The athlete or his representative then checks the written information on the form and signs a copy which is also signed by the official. The samples are then sent off with documentation to the testing laboratory. There are no details on the form that will identify the sample as coming from any particular athlete and therefore the laboratory testing these samples is totally blind.

The laboratory will test sample A and if it is found positive, it informs the drug testing authorities who inform the competitor. The competitor or his representative are entitled to be present at the unsealing and testing of sample B, which if it also proves positive will mean that the sporting organisation is informed. It is the sporting organisation that applies the penalty, usually after a hearing with the athlete and his representative.

It is important that the athlete's representative supports the athlete throughout this process and observes the process taking place. It is not only to ensure that the correct procedure is followed but also that the facilities are available.

If the athlete is charged with an offence and given a penalty there is an appeals procedure, during which it is important for the athlete to be aware whether the testing procedure was carried out correctly in all details, and whether the penalty appears to be just.

ROLE OF THE TEAM DOCTOR

The role of the team physician is extremely important in prevention and management of doping issues within sport. It is therefore important that a team physician should be up-to-date and totally familiar with all issues relating to drug doping. He should also educate all members of the team, including management and coaches and especially players, and this should involve regular meetings and presentations especially prior to the season.

Within this remit, the physician should make sure that all athletes under his care are familiar with the doping process, and the responsibilities that they have for a drug-free sport. He should also know exactly which medications, whether prescribed or otherwise, each athlete is on and arrange for the submission of a TUE for the athlete if appropriate (see below). The physician should inform all players that over-the-counter medications and supplements may not be 'safe' and certainly in a survey of freely available supplements that were not meant to have any banned substances, almost 25% were found to have traces of banned substances.[14] The athlete needs to be made aware that the processes by which a supplement is produced is very different to the quality control processes by which a drug medication is produced and therefore cross-contamination from banned substances may occur when used in the same manufacturing process. The physician also needs to inform athletes when travelling abroad, that similar names for drugs may not necessarily mean similar contents and ingredients, and that they should always check their medication with the physician before taking it. It is important to emphasise that the responsibility of taking medications, and its consequences lies solely with the athlete. It is also important, at this stage, for the physician to emphasise the importance of not taking drugs, not only because of the risk of penalising, but to keep sport safe. As mentioned previously, athletes are under constant pressure to improve performance and it is the role of the team physician to reinforce this ethos. Primarily it is the role of the sports physician to consider the health of the athlete and the adverse effect of drugs on him, and that he has a confidentiality issue and a medical ethics issue in his relationship with the athlete. It is important to remember that a doctor's main responsibility is to treat those players who are ill and enable them to compete up to their normal training levels during a competition without risk of further injury. It is not an uncommon scenario where an athlete may ask a doctor to give him a pain-killing injection to allow him to compete. The injection may be permitted under wider rules and in practice, but even an injection may not allow an athlete to compete to their maximum ability. However, the main question is whether or not an injection is likely to produce injury or further damage to the athlete. The factors involved in this include: experience of the athlete, his age and past experience of injection, the length of time before competition and the type and site of injury. The ultimate decision lies with the athlete after informed discussion and as long as the doctor is not condoning the use of banned substances or putting the athlete at further risk, there may be a role for giving an injection as long as there is informed consent. The decision obviously lies with each individual, but like most ethical dilemmas, there is no clear-cut answer. Another dilemma may occur when an athlete seeks medical opinion from a team physician, asking about the pros and cons of taking performance-enhancing drugs to improve his performance. It may be that the athlete is sourcing these drugs from alternative areas but such a question highlights several issues: what is the doctor's role in preventing drug abuse, how does this affect the doctor/patient relationship and is there any indication to break confidentiality and inform others? Again, with ethical dilemmas there are various responses to these questions; however, the specific physician needs to be sure that he is primarily the athlete's physician and that he should advise the athlete as he would in a normal patient/doctor relationship, respecting individuality and confidentiality. It may be that the physician might need advice from his medical defence union; however, there is a role for the physician here in opening up discussion with the athlete, by asking why he would want to take banned medication when the risks of detection are high and the penalties severe. Likewise, he should explore the pressures the athlete is under that are making him feel he needs to take this risk and also whether he is aware of the significant side-effects that may have short- or long-term effects on his health. Finally, it may be appropriate at this time to educate the athlete on the permitted options including nutrition, psychology and training methods that may help him improve his performance legitimately. The team physician can help him facilitate this by coordinating the discussion with the coach.

Finally, it is important to make sure that each athlete is aware of the significant risks of inadvertent violation of the doping regulations by taking over-the-counter medications. Most pharmacists should have access, via the BNF (British National Formulary) to identify which drugs are on the banned list; however, if you have a good rapport with your athletes, it would be helpful if they discussed with you whether it is safe to take a medication before they actually do.

Therapeutic use exemption (TUE) forms

As mentioned previously, there may be genuine medical reasons why an athlete may need to take banned substances to keep him healthy. These may include: inhaled beta agonists for asthma; inhaled glucocorticosteroids for asthma or hay fever control; oral glucocorticosteroids for suppression of inflammatory conditions such as colitis; insulin therapy for diabetics; diuretics for the management of hypertension and congestive cardiac failure; erythropoietin for anaemia due to renal failure; tamoxifen for breast cancer. Doctors have a role in confirming the presence of these medical conditions and informing WADA so that no discrepancies occur. TUE forms may be completed by the physician and the athlete confirming the medical condition and the treatment regime, and on what basis the diagnosis was made. The criteria by which a TUE form can be completed include:

- The athlete would experience significant health problems without taking the prohibited substance.
- The use of the substances in therapeutic doses would not produce significant enhancement of performance.
- There is no other reasonable therapeutic treatment other than the prohibited substance.

There are two types of form: there is a *standard TUE form*, which needs to be completed for all medications other than glucocorticosteroids used by non-systemic routes and beta 2 agonists by the inhalation routes. The process by which a standard TUE is completed is as follows: the physician and athlete complete the form and submit it to the chief medical officer of the sporting association or sporting organisation. With this form there needs to be complementary documentation from the specialist physician who confirms the diagnosis, and the method by which this diagnosis was made, and the treatment regime which cannot be substituted by any other form. Once this form has been submitted, the athlete needs to receive an authorisation notice from the organisation before starting the medication. This form needs to be renewed and submitted on an annual basis.

The other form of TUE is an inhaled beta 2 agonist TUE for use of inhaled salbutamol or long-acting beta 2 agonist for treatment of asthma. These have recently superseded the abbreviated TUE forms. In these forms, the physician completing the form needs to supply documented evidence of airflow limitation at rest which is then corrected by the inhalation of bronchodilators. This is shown via spirometry readings of forced vital capacity (FVC) and forced expiratory volume in 1 s (FEV1). Evidence of airflow limitation is confirmed by a resting FEV1 of less than 80% predicted and a positive bronchodilator challenge test of the FEV1 increasing by more than 12% from baseline after short-acting beta 2 agonist inhalation. If neither of these can provide evidence of airflow limitation then an EVH or mannitol challenge test is required.

Glucocorticoids administered by either inhalation or localised injection (e.g. peri- or intra-articular injection) do not require a TUE but should be notified via a declaration of use form accessed on-line via the 100% ME website.

Take home points

- As a team physician, know the difference in procedures between the different types of TUE and declaration forms.
- WADA produce an updated list of prohibited drugs on 1 January every year.
- Know the drug testing procedure.

 CLINICAL CASE

You attend as team physician to a rugby team as the representative of a player who has been notified to attend for drug testing at the end of a rugby game. The procedure is completed in the correct manner with the correct facilities, witnessed by you as team physician, and everything goes to plan until the final completion of the form. The athlete has completed the form stating he is on no medication and has not taken anything over the last 7 days, and is just about to sign the declaration at the end of the form to complete the process when he looks up and asks you as team physician for some advice. In the presence of the drug testing officer he asks you what he should do. He then relays the story that 2 days previously he was at a dinner party with his wife, together with other couples. After the meal there was coffee and biscuits together with a cake the host had made. He tells you he thought nothing of it and ate two pieces of cake and returned home after an enjoyable evening. The next day he was informed by the host of the party that the cake he had made contained cannabis. The player now asks you as team physician whether you should declare that he took cannabis, knowing that if he did there would potentially be a 2-year ban.

What do you advise the player to do?

This example raises several issues that include the responsibility and education of players being aware that drugs can be administered to them in various forms.

This situation could have been avoided, if the player had come to you before the game and together you had gone to the coach stating that there was a risk that he could have inadvertently taken cannabis, and therefore be at risk of being banned. It may well be that his selection for the rugby game could have been avoided and cannabis being an in-competition test only, would mean that he would not have been banned if he had been found to be positive out of competition. Finally, what do you do as sports physician in terms of advising this player? If you advise him to amend the form to say that he has taken cannabis, then you may be undermining the drug-testing process and be seen to be colluding with the player in avoiding detection.

My advice to the player here is that if there is the possibility that he has inadvertently ingested cannabis, and that it will be detected in the drug-testing process, then he should declare this on the form, however, he should also declare on the form that it was an inadvertent ingestion and explain the situation by which it occurred. The reason for this is that if he is found positive, then it will come to a hearing, and if he is seen to have admitted to it and the process by which it got into his system at the testing point of the procedure, then the sporting organisation may look more favourably on his penalty.

Whatever your personal feelings as team physician as to how this came about, it is important that you support the player and advise him as appropriately as you see fit. Although it is not easy on the drug-testing form to write any details, if you as a physician or as a player feel that there is extra documentation you need to include, this should be included.

REFERENCES

1. Yesalis CE, Herrick RT, Buckley WE et al. Self-reported use of anabolic-androgenic steroids by elite power lifters. Phys Sportsmed 1988; 16(12):91–98.
2. International Olympic Committee Anti-Doping Rules. Chateau de Vidy, CP 356, CH-1007 Lausanne, Switzerland.
3. WADA. List of Banned Substances. Online. Available: www.wada-ama.org
4. Moran A, Guerin S, MacIntyre T, McCaffery N. Why do athletes cheat? An investigation of Irish athletes' understanding of, and attitudes to, cheating behaviour (including doping), in sport. Final report to the Irish Sports Council, 2004.
5. Lindström M, Nilsson AL, Katzman PL et al. Use of anabolic-androgenic steroids among body builders – frequency and attitudes. J Intern Med 1990; 227(6):407–411.
6. Giorgi A, Weatherby RP, Murphy PW. Muscular strength, body composition and health responses to the use of testosterone enanthate: a double blind study. J Sci Med Sport 1999; 2(4):341–355.
7. Pärssinen M, Seppälä T. Steroid use and longterm health risks in former athletes. Sports Med 2002; 32(2): 83–94.
8. Ishak KG, Zimmerman HJ. Hepatotoxic effects of the anabolic/androgenic steroids. Semin Liver Dis 1987; 7(3):230–236.
9. Choi PYL, Parrott AC, Cowan D. Adverse behavioural effects of anabolic steroids in athletes: a brief review. Clin Sports Med 1989; 1:183–187.
10. Scott J, Phillips GC. Erythropoietin in sports: a new look at an old problem. Curr Sports Med Rep 2005; 4(4):224–226.
11. Corrigan B. Beyond EPO. Clin J Sports Med 2002; 12(4):242–244.
12. Rennie MJ. Claims for the anabolic effects of growth hormone: a case of the emperor's new clothes? Br J Sports Med 2003; 37(2):100–105.
13. Seehusen DA, Glorioso JE. Tamoxifen as an ergogenic agent in women body-builders. A case report. Clin J Sports Med 2002; 12(5):313–314.
14. Sandomir R. Olympics: Banned substances found in many food supplements. New York Times 12.10.01.

Chapter | 5 |

Musculoskeletal injury

© 2009 Elsevier Ltd, Inc, BV
DOI: 10.1016/B978-0-443-06813-3.00008-9

Injuries to musculoskeletal structures can be divided into two main groups; those due to acute injuries and those due to overuse injuries. Both injuries may have a brief history of onset as regards their symptoms and signs; however, an acute injury may not be attributable to a developing pathology and occurs out of the blue, such as a bone fracture or a tear within a muscle. Overuse injuries, however, may have a more gradual onset and a multifactorial cause, whether it be related to training load, biomechanics, previous injury or inadequate rehabilitation. This may predispose to an injury that may present over a chronic period of time or may be sub-clinical and then present with an acute onset. The following text will describe different types of acute and overuse injuries affecting the musculoskeletal system and summarise their symptoms, signs and treatment.

ACUTE INJURIES

Injuries to bone

The bones provide a rigid structure to the skeleton and are a site of rigid attachment of muscles, tendons and ligaments. It also provides protection to vulnerable soft tissues within the skeleton. Activity increases the strength of bone and thickens the structure, whereas inactivity weakens them. Bones can adapt to stress applied to them as long as the stress is applied gradually. An acute stress or dramatic increase in the stress results in fracture. Bones are better at resisting compression rather than tension or torsion and that is why fractures mostly occur on torsional forces.

A fracture may occur either as a result of a direct blow as in trauma or as a result of indirect trauma such as a torsional injury. Fractures may be transverse, oblique, spiral or comminuted and a special group in adolescents exists as a form of avulsion, where a tendon or ligament that is stronger than the piece of bone to which it is attached pulls the fragment away from the bone. Fractures may result in distortion of the bone in terms of angulation, rotation and shortening and the aim of treatment is to return the fractured bones as precisely as possible to their correct position and reduce any malalignment. Some fractures are more common in certain sports, such as tibial fractures in soccer players, forearm fractures in gymnasts and clavicular fractures in horse riders.

Features of a fracture include swelling and progressive bruising in the injured area and tenderness and pain at the site of injury, aggravated by loading the limb and movement of the injured site, deformity and abnormal mobility of the limb and restriction of movement. Occasionally, these symptoms are lessened when there is a compression injury such as in the neck of the femur, where signs may be minimal.

Treatment includes: first aid measures, such as covering the open injury with a sterile compress and clean bandage; immobilising the limb by splinting or bracing; elevating the injured limb; and arranging further investigation and transport to hospital for imaging. It is important to confirm the presence of vascular or neurological impairment at an early stage to prevent any ischaemia or long-term nerve damage. The correction of malalignment or the relocation of a dislocated joint on site when there may be vascular or neurological deficit can be limb-saving. It is important to document exactly the sequence of events and to be sure of your actions for medico–legal reasons.

Non-displaced fractures can be treated by immobilisation in a cast, boot or brace with advice for the patient to be aware of increased pain, swelling and/or tingling distal to the calves that may be signs of compartment syndrome. Bracing will help the fracture heal but will result in stiffness of the joint above and below the brace, and, therefore, following removal of the brace active mobilisation needs to occur.

Displaced fractures need to be realigned either by manipulation or with fixation, and then immobilised.

Complications of fractures include infection, which is most likely to occur in open fractures, acute compartment syndrome where rapid swelling of the muscle compartment around the fracture causes a rise in pressure within the fascial sheath and ischaemia, not only of the muscle, but of the distal structures including the nerves and blood vessels. The patient complains of severe pain, usually at the fracture site or distal to the fracture site, which may be out of proportion to the degree of initial injury associated with pallor, paraesthesia and pulselessness and pain on passive stretching (all the 'Ps'). This requires urgent recognition and decompression with fasciotomy as a medical emergency.

Other complications include injury to associated structures such as muscles, ligaments, tendons, nerves and blood vessels. Certain fractures have a close proximity to these structures, including distal humerus and the brachial artery and median nerve, distal radius and the median nerve and olecranon fractures and the ulna nerve. Specifically, neck of femur and scaphoid fractures may result in avascular necrosis due to their unique blood supply and the importance of this needs to be recognised. Further complications include deep vein thrombosis as a result of immobilisation of lower limb fractures and its subsequent pulmonary embolism, as well as fat embolisms of long bone fractures and pelvic fractures. Do not under-estimate the degree of haemorrhage that may occur as a result of a fracture, mainly within the long bones but especially in the pelvis, and the shock and hypotension that can quickly ensue.

Other complications include delayed and non-union of fractures as well as mal-union. In adolescents, injury to the growth plate can be a complication as classified by the Salter–Harris classification where Grades 1 and 2 can be treated conservatively but Grades 3, 4 and 5 need special consideration and possibly orthopaedic surgical intervention. The risk of injury to the growth plate can result in asymmetrical growth and lead to malalignment and disproportionate growth within joints and long-term complications. Avulsion fractures are unique to the adolescent age group and do not need surgical correction unless there is a signifi-cant fragment or displacement. Most can be treated with conservative therapy.

Articular cartilage injury

The articular cartilage is the smooth, shiny covering on the ends of the long bones that allows smooth movement of the joints by reducing friction and pro-viding protection for the bones through shock absorption. The articular cartilage lacks any vascular, nerve or lymphatic supply and as a result has limited tissue repair capacity and is dependent on the exchange of synovial fluid for nutrients and oxygen. The cartilage is made up of chondrocytes which produce a matrix of collagen and proteoglycans which attract water into the cartilage providing 70% of its total volume. On weight-bearing, the water content is compressed back out into the joint hence the shock absorbance effect. The lack of nerve supply means that injuries to the articular cartilage may be pain free. Injuries may occur acutely due to trauma injuring the articular cartilage but also can occur slowly as a form of repetitive small injures causing 'wear and tear' injuries that may progress to osteoarthritis. Acute and minor injuries to the articular car-tilage are more commonly diagnosed now due to the imaging techniques of MRI and increasing availability of arthroscopy. Asymptomatic lesions are increasingly being diagnosed in arthroscopy. The importance of diagnosing these lesions is primarily that they can progress to further damage of the joint and osteoarthritis. Injuries can occur by dislocation, contusion and compression of a joint and malalignment of a joint can be a contributing factor for repeated micro trauma.

There have been several grading classifications of articular cartilage injuries and these follow two formats.

The first classification is defined by the depth of the lesion, usually best seen on imaging, and is divided into:

1. Superficial or partial, where a maximum of 50% of the depth of the cartilage is injured or deficient. These do not heal but can progress to a more serious injury.
2. Deep or complete, where there is an injury down to the subchondral bone but not through it. Likewise, these do not heal but can progress to osteoarthritis.
3. Osteochondral injuries, where there is injury down and through the subchondral bone to the trabecular bone. These can heal as the bone has a vascular supply and will fill in with fibroblast producing a fibrous scar.

Alternatively, grading can be made according to the arthroscopic appearance as follows:

1. Fissures extending into the superficial layer of the cartilage
2. Increased injury into the cartilage with multiple fissures but not down to subchondral bone

3. Worsening fissures down into the subchondral bone but not exposing the subchondral bone

4. Complete loss of the cartilage exposing the subchondral bone.

The symptoms of articular cartilage injuries depend on the site, the most common lesion areas being the articular surfaces of the talus, femoral condyles, patella and capitellum of the humerus. The patient may present with a history of distortion or dislocation and there may be swelling or bleeding or an effusion of a joint. Pain is precipitated by movement of the joint and there may be a catching or locking feeling on joint movement. Crepitus may be heard or felt.

The physician needs to have a high index of suspicion for osteochondral lesions and progress to imaging with a view to arthroscopy. Acutely, the bleeding within the joint can be drained and cleaned out and removal or fixing of the osteochondral fragment can be beneficial. In chronic situations where this has occurred over a gradual period of time, MRI scans can give an idea of whether the fragment is stable or unstable. A stable lesion is one where there is Grade 1 or 2 classification with no evidence of any fluid-filled cleft beneath the fragment that may imply that it is going to become dislodged. A Grade 3 or 4 lesion would suggest instability and will need arthroscopy. A stable lesion will require 6 weeks of low-impact rest or non-weight-bearing rest with a range of movement exercises and strengthening exercises followed by a graded rehabilitation programme. Unstable lesions require arthroscopy where debridement of loose cartilage is followed by drilling, microfracturing or abrasion of the defect. The idea of this is to encourage trauma to the subchondral bone which bleeds into the defect creating a fibrous repair. If this is unsuccessful, then further tissue engineering with either autologous chondrocyte transplantation or perichondrial and periosteal grafting may be indicated. The recovery from this is slow, as there is a significant period of several months of non-weight-bearing; however, some grafting results have been promising.

 ## Joint dislocation

An acute dislocation or subluxation of a joint occurs when there is loss of continuity of articular surfaces of a joint in trauma. It is important to realise before rushing back into relocating a joint that injury to the surrounding structures can occur as has already been mentioned, such as injuries to blood vessels, nerves, tendons and ligaments, as well as avulsion fractures and articular cartilage injuries. Ideally all dislocations should be imaged before relocation; however, urgent relocation may need to be performed before this if there is imminent and progressive damage to the nerves or vascular supply where time is of the essence to relocate the joint. It is important to confirm relocation of the joint with further imaging and to document the vascular and neurological deficit as well as injuries to tendons and ligaments for medico–legal reasons.

Symptoms suggestive of dislocation include pain on movement, abnormal contour of the joint, swelling and tenderness within the joint and instability of the joint.

Ligamentous injuries

Ligaments provide stability to a joint, together with the joint capsule. Both are made of connective tissue and the capsule is thickened at points of stress to form a ligament. Ligaments are not contractile tissue but provide an end-point to extreme range of motion. When a joint is moved beyond its normal range of movement or a load is applied to it that is excessive, then the ligament fails and tears rather than causing injury to the attached bone. Ligament injuries are graded one to three depending on the amount of fibres within the ligament that are damaged. The greater the number of fibres the higher the instability of the joint as a result.

Grade 1 ligament injuries represent only disruption of a few fibres and stretching of some others and clinical examination shows the normal range of movement on stressing the ligament with no laxity although there may be some pain.

Grade 2 injury involves disruption of more than 50% of the fibres resulting in increased instability of the joint and examination will reveal increased laxity on stressing the ligament but there will be a definite end point to feel.

Grade 3 tears represent complete disruption of all the fibres as in a rupture. Examination will reveal excessive joint laxity with no firm end point. Ironically, Grade 3 injuries are often less painful or pain free as the sensory fibres within the ligament are often divided during the injury.

The patient may sustain a valgus or varus injury to the joint associated with bruising, swelling and tenderness along the joint line. The ligament itself may be tender on palpation and most noticeable is the degree of instability or laxity of the joint on stress testing.

   Management involves the RICE regime with support, possibly a brace. Grades 1 and 2 injuries involve conservative treatment including electrotherapeutic modalities, joint mobilisation and soft tissue massage to promote tissue healing, prevent joint stiffness and protect against further damage. Recovery can be anything from 10 days to 2 months, depending on the severity of the injury. Rehabilitation involving strength, stability and proprioception are vitally important. Grade 3 ruptures used to require surgical reconstruction as well as bracing; however, there is a movement towards bracing and conservative treatment, especially involving the medial collateral ligament of the knee. Some ligaments, however, are not amenable to primary surgical repair and require a graft, such as the ACL which can be grafted with hamstring, patella tendon or donor grafts.

 ## Tendon injuries

Tendon injuries are often forgotten or misdiagnosed and are generally not managed as well as other acute injuries. They tend to occur at points of poor blood supply and a resistance to high forces at its weakest and this may be complicated by the presence of tendinopathy at the same site. Complete or partial tendon ruptures may occur when a tension is applied quickly and sustained without adequate warm up or when the tension is applied obliquely. They can also occur when a muscle group is stretched by external forces or when the tendon is weak in comparison to the muscle as occurs in tendinopathy. Tendon injury can occur as a result of trauma to the bone in the form of fracture or dislocation and attention needs to be given to this, especially tendon ruptures with the interphalangeal joint dislocation where all the attention is taken by the bone dislocation and rupture of flexor or extensor tendons is often missed.

   Most notably, however, tendon ruptures can occur and the two most common ruptured tendons are the Achilles tendon and the supraspinatus tendon in the shoulder. Complete ruptures are most commonly treated with surgical repair although some Achilles ruptures are treated conservatively. Partial tears can mimic tendinopathy and the two can coexist; however, a good history and imaging will reveal the diagnosis.

Muscle injuries

Muscle injuries can exist in two forms, either as a strain or tear or as a contusion or haematoma. Tears occur when the muscle fibres fail to cope with the overstretching or eccentric overload put onto them. This occurs most commonly in the musculotendinous junction and usually occurs when there is changeover between the eccentric and concentric contraction of the muscle that occurs during explosive muscular effort. Tears more commonly affect a muscle that spans two joints, such as the hamstrings, the rectus femoris of the quadriceps and the gastrocnemius muscle. This is because the muscles cannot perform two functions at the same time that are governed by a sensitive neuromuscular system. Other factors that predispose to muscle strains include inadequate warm-up and preparation of the muscle, and previous injury to a muscle involving inadequate rehabilitation; however, even muscles that have been adequately rehabilitated are at more risk of injury as can be seen by recurrent hamstring injuries. Muscles that are fatigued, overused or have inadequate recovery, muscles that are excessively tight or have faulty biomechanics as well as those who have muscle imbalance and therefore are consequently overloaded, are at risk. Muscles that have inadequate neuromuscular input such as those with neurological or spinal dysfunction are also at risk.

Like ligaments, muscle strains and tears can be classified into three grades:

Grade 1 strains involve a small number of muscle fibres and although they may be tender show full range of movement and no loss of strength.

Grade 2 tears result in a significant number of muscle fibres being damaged which results in increasing pain and swelling and limited range of movement with pain on resisted muscle contraction. Power is reduced and range of movement is limited by pain.

Grade 3 strains or complete ruptures of the muscle may reveal proximal retraction of the muscle belly with a palpable defect and no ability to contract against resistance.

The patient may complain of a sharp or stabbing pain at the moment of injury that is reproduced on resisted contraction of the muscle. The severity of the injury can be diagnosed clinically as listed above but, often, imaging is required to be absolutely sure.

Management of the muscle strains requires first aid to minimise bleeding, swelling and inflammation and subsequent treatment promotes efficient scar formation through the use of strengthening exercises, soft tissue therapy and stretching. Adequate strengthening exercises as well as addressing biomechanical and postural defects are important to prevent recurrence.

Muscle contusions and haematomas

A direct impact on a muscle causes a contusion resulting in injury, rupture and bleeding deep within the muscle fibres. Direct impacts are most common in collision sports and most commonly occur at the front of the thigh and the quadriceps muscle. They are otherwise known as 'corks' or 'Charlie Horse'. During activity the blood supply to the muscles is vast and when a muscle is damaged a significant amount of bleeding occurs. A haematoma can develop between the muscle groups when a muscle fascia and its blood vessels are damaged. This is known as intermuscular haematoma. On these occasions, the bleeding that occurs disperses quickly within the fascial layers and typically bruising and swelling appear distally to the damaged area within 48 h of the injury, caused by gravity. There is no increased pressure within the muscle group and swelling is temporary and muscle function is rapidly restored. Conversely, if haematoma is confined within a muscle group, this is called an intramuscular haematoma. Swelling can occur within a muscle itself and is accompanied by tenderness, pain and impaired mobility. There is often less bruising and muscle function can be dramatically impaired. In an acute situation this can lead to acute compartment syndrome although this is rare.[1]

Management of a contusion involves minimising the bleeding and swelling and historically this has involved rest, icing, compression and elevation. Evidence suggests, however, that compression with the muscle on a stretch, such as keeping the knee flexed, may encourage the dispersal of the haematoma and a more rapid return to play.

The patient may complain of acute pain within a muscle group and the muscle itself may be totally dysfunctional requiring the player to come off the pitch. Quite rapidly there may be reduction in range of movement, and a reduction of knee flexion to less than 90° may imply an intramuscular haematoma. The importance of an intramuscular haematoma not only signifies a more prolonged recovery programme but these haematomas are at risk of complication in the form of myositis ossificans. This occurs when a haematoma calcifies and is most common following intramuscular haematomas. They are also more common when a haematoma is subjected to massage within the first 48–72 h of a muscular injury and therefore massage should not be used. Myositis ossificans should be suspected in a muscle contusion that does not resolve in a normal time frame. It may be diagnosed either by X-ray, which shows calcification, or at an earlier stage by ultrasound, which can also show organisation of the haematoma with calcification. Management of myositis ossificans is conservative and is felt to be due to the presence of osteoblasts and osteoclasts within the haematoma that try to form bone within the haematoma itself. Generally, the haematoma is more painful and enlarges and can cause nerve impingement on surrounding nerves. The management is conservative and avoidance of further trauma by offloading and protecting the area. Early surgical excision can be counterproductive in that this can reform and cause further problems. Treatment involving bisphosphonates has had limited success in some studies. Return to sport can occur when the area is no longer tender and the muscle has regained its full function. This can take up to 8 weeks.

OVERUSE INJURIES

As mentioned above, overuse injuries occur more chronically when the load on the musculoskeletal structure is progressive and repetitively outweighs the tensile strength of the structure itself. Although these conditions can present acutely, they usually represent a gradual history and good history taking can reveal this. A cause for all overuse injuries should be found, as without this, the condition may recur. Generally speaking, overuse injuries are caused by extrinsic or intrinsic factors and these include:

Extrinsic factors – changes in training load including volume, intensity, surface and inadequate recovery. Faulty technique or equipment, including shoes and footwear, as well as training in extreme environmental conditions.

Intrinsic factors – involve biomechanical abnormalities such as leg length discrepancies and malalignment, including rearfoot varus, genu valgum and patella alta (among others), muscle imbalance and muscle weakness as well as loss of flexibility.

As a general rule of thumb, training load should not increase by more than 10% a week to prevent an overuse injury.

History and examination should include exploring the above factors, and management involves relative rest, avoiding the aggravating precipitating factors, reducing pain and relative inflammation, correcting the predisposing factor and reducing inflammation with soft tissue techniques and medication such as antiinflammatories or cortisone injections. Overuse injuries affecting parts of the musculoskeletal system include the following.

Bone

Stress fractures are the most common bony overuse injury and represent a spectrum from normal bone structure through stress reaction to stress fracture to occult fracture. Overloading torsional forces on the bone to a level where the bone is not able to compensate results in weakening of the trabeculae and microfracture causing bleeding within the honeycomb architecture of the bone. This is visible on MRI scans as bone oedema and bruising, and has an area of increased uptake on isotope bone scans. Further stress on the bone may result in fractures within the trabecular bone that may extend to the cortex and these are therefore defined as stress fractures. If there is still further loading on the bone then the cortex fracture can extend to result in a traumatic fracture. This, therefore, represents a spectrum of reaction of the bone to increasing load. Stress fractures occur at sites of maximum stress or sites of poor bone nutrition and there are several bones within the skeleton particularly vulnerable to a stress fracture, both in their occurrence and in their ability to heal. The most common bones affected are the tibia, metatarsals, femur and pelvis but stress fractures of the 5th metatarsal, the navicular and talus bone as well as the neck of the femur are particularly vulnerable to non-union or avascular necrosis and need to be defined as high risk stress fractures. These require specific treatment other than outlined below and further details on their management can be found in the Common injures part of the enclosed DVD.[2]

The patient may complain of insidious onset of exercise-related pain. Initially, the symptoms of pain are felt during activity but not at rest following a change in training load. The pain initially may settle after activity but with increasing training the pain increases in intensity and may exist as a dull ache persisting many hours after exercise. The pain is often worse on impact and can be felt at night. Occasionally, there will be local swelling and tenderness over the fracture site. Specific bony tenderness on examination is a common finding in stress fractures. Early investigation with isotope bone scan, MRI or CT scans will show increased uptake or hot spots and are preferable to X-rays which may show no abnormality within the first 4 weeks. Management of stress fractures requires offloading and the avoidance of the precipitating activity. The majority of fractures heal within 6 weeks, once relative rest is started. Monitoring of a stress fracture does not involve repeated imaging but is assessed clinically by the presence of local tenderness and the ability of the athlete to perform a precipitating activity without pain. Once the patient is no longer tender on palpation and able to perform a progressive exercise regime involving walking, cross-training, hopping and running symptom free then they are able to progress to a graded running programme. During this 6-week programme, the precipitating factors need to be addressed together with the diet of the athlete to include adequate calcium intake as well as a high carbohydrate intake that provides support for the 'fatiguing' bone. Low frequency ultrasound treatment in the form of Exogen therapy has been shown to enhance bone healing in stress fractures in as much as 38% in some cases.[3] A bone densitometry scan may be indicated in those at risk such as female athletes with a history of eating disorders and amenorrhoea.

Muscle

Overuse conditions of the muscle mainly include chronic compartment syndromes. These usually affect the muscles of the lower limb but in rowers, throwers and racquet players can affect the muscles of the upper limb. Muscles of the limbs are divided into different compartments surrounded by fascia. If the fascia layer is tight then the muscle is unable to expand adequately during exercise. As a result the pressure within the muscle group increases and reaches a level which impairs the vascular supply to that muscle. The muscle, therefore, becomes relatively ischaemic causing pain, discomfort, dysfunction of the muscle and sometimes impairment of the distal neurological supply as the nerve through the muscle also becomes impaired. Often the pain is so severe that the athlete has to stop activity and, as a result, the pressure within the fascial sheath falls, the vascular supply improves and the pain subsides. This can occur within 20 min of stopping the activity.

The patient therefore complains of an exercise-related muscle pain, sometimes with an associated muscle pain, sometimes with an associated distal paraesthesia or numbness. The muscle group may feel tense and tight and bulging and may have small herniations through the fascial sheath that are visible. Classically there are no symptoms at rest or at night but they can be anticipated with a set degree of activity. This is useful in examining the patient after exercise and diagnosis can be made by compartment pressure testing.

Conservative treatment has a limited role in the form of deep tissue massage, biomechanical correction, muscle strengthening and stretching as well as acupuncture to the fascial sheath. Definitive treatment, however, is surgical in the form of fasciotomy or fasciectomy. The latter is preferable to prevent healing of the fascia and scarring resulting in a recurrence of the condition.

Tendon

Overuse injuries of the tendon are called tendinopathies. No longer do we use the term tendonitis as histological samples of these conditions confirm that there are no inflammatory cells present. Collagen fibre failure within the tendon occurs when the stress on the tendon increases and this is located at sites of vulnerable vascular supply, most commonly 2 inches proximal to the Achilles tendon insertion and over the articular surface of the supraspinatus tendon in the shoulder. The proximal portion of the patella tendon at the inferior pole of the patella and the common extensor origin of the extensor tendons are also common sites.[4]

Clinically, these patients present with a gradual onset of pain and tenderness over the tendon with swelling and pain on resisted activity. Classically, they present as an 'inflammatory' picture. It is important to be aware that tendinopathies can not only occur with overuse activities but are associated with other generalised inflammatory conditions such as spondyloarthropathy, gout, psoriasis and rheumatological diseases. Imaging of the tendons can be seen best with dynamic ultrasound where there is degeneration and tears within the tendon associated with neovascularisation. It is unclear what the neovascularisation represents but initially it was felt to be a guide to the degree of pain the patient was suffering, and therefore, obliterating the neovascularisation would help with pain, and certainly some studies show that the neovascularisation decreases once this is treated. However, this is not always the case. Management of tendinopathy is a prolonged process and evidence-based treatment includes exercise therapy in the form of eccentric strengthening exercises. These need to be progressive and with high volume as this has been shown to help alignment and recovery of the collagen fibres within the tendon. Other forms of treatment include nitrous oxide patches, sclerosant injections, dry needling and autologous blood injections. This is used in conjunction with relative rest, electrotherapeutic modalities and soft tissue therapies. Return to sport involves a progressive reloading programme, correction of biomechanics and the other overload issues that have precipitated the injury followed by a dedicated rehabilitation programme.

MANAGEMENT OF ACUTE MUSCULOSKELETAL INJURIES

In this section, the management of acute musculoskeletal injuries is going to be divided into two parts: the first part deals with what can be described as pitch-side or emergency management and the second part deals with subsequent management, which involves treatment beyond the first hour of an injury.

Pitch-side or emergency treatment

There are several fully validated and affiliated courses solely in the management of acute injuries on the pitch side and the reader is thoroughly recommended to enrol on these courses, not only to provide more detailed knowledge than this book can provide, but also to give useful hands-on experience in the moulages of these courses. However, a summary of what can be regarded as a check-list to use as a framework for immediate management care is provided as follows.[5]

The phrase 'DR ABCDES' outlines the titles that you need to cover in this specific order, so as not only not to miss any stage but also not to do one stage out of sync with the others.

Danger

Before entering any emergency situation, be it on a rugby pitch or assisting someone in a Formula 1 accident, you need to make sure that there is no danger to yourself and that it is safe to enter the arena. This can include not interfering with the run of play or putting yourself at risk from explosives or injury from other vehicles or players. Different sports have different rules about entering the field of play with or without the referee's permission and the attending physician needs to be aware of the rules before running onto a pitch. Safety also includes safety for the health of the therapist and this includes risk of infection from open wounds and blood-borne diseases as well as risk of infection, although very slim, from mouth-to-mouth resuscitation. The wearing of protective gloves and the practice of covering wounds and using masks or artificial airways to assist in resuscitation have reduced this risk.

Response

On arriving at the patient's side it is important to assess the level of consciousness and the response to commands from the player. The therapist may have an idea of this as he is running towards the player as he may see the player talking or responding to other players. It is probably not advisable, however, to start shaking an unconscious player to see if they respond, as they may also have a neck injury, so simple commands such as: 'Can you hear me?' or 'Open your eyes', may be all that is needed. If the player opens his eyes to command and starts speaking to you then you immediately know his level of alertness and also some assessment of his airway and breathing situation. However, if there is no response, then likewise you know that you are going to need more help and it is at this stage that you ask for further assistance from your colleagues, the referee or on-site paramedics.

In a traumatic injury one should immediately assume a cervical spine injury and although this is not the most important element of resuscitation nor one that you address immediately, it is an area that you need to be aware of and can address while assessing the other factors. In other words, if you can secure the neck and fix it while assessing other areas, or ideally get a colleague to fix the neck while you are assessing other areas, then this is preferential. All others areas are assessed with the knowledge that a cervical spine injury may have occurred.

Airway

The airway is the most important element to assess and must be assessed before anything else. If the patient is talking they have a good airway but they may be unconscious and assessing an open airway can be difficult. Looking out for grunting or snoring can suggest airway obstruction and immediately the airway needs to be opened with a jaw-thrust if a cervical spine is suspected, otherwise a head-tilt and chin lift may be adequate. Although this may be adequate to open the airway, it is possible that suction may be required or removal of loose fragments or teeth. Well-fitting dentures should remain in site if not obstructing the airway. If there is a suspicion that the airway may be further compromised, then an oropharyngeal or nasopharyngeal airway should be inserted. The latter is not inserted if there is evidence of a facial or base of skull fracture.

Breathing

Once the airway has been secured, assessment of the breathing needs to be performed. This is done by looking, listening and feeling – the rise and fall of the chest and movement of the diaphragm is watched for, the noise of respiration is listened for and the movement of air in and out of the mouth or nose is felt for on the examiner's cheek. Once it has been determined that the player is breathing, then the assessment of breathing needs to be further analysed in terms of whether it is adequate to maintain ventilation. Examination at this stage of the level of expiration, respiratory rate, air entry and breath sounds within the chest accompanied by percussion note and dilation of chest veins can give some idea of whether both lungs are being ventilated adequately and if not, whether there is any unilateral lung disease that may compromise ventilation. Assisted ventilation can be provided by a pocket mask or mouth-to-mouth resuscitation, where 15% oxygen is supplemented into the patient. However, a re-breathe bag or bag valve mask system is preferred with 60% oxygen, or ideally an ET tube inserted if the therapist has the adequate skills and this can provide 85% oxygen. It is important at this stage to exclude any airway obstruction such as laryngeal injury that may require a needle cricothyroidotomy or any potentially life-threatening chest trauma such as a tension pneumothorax, open pneumothorax or haemothorax, flailed chest or cardiac tamponade that would need action at this stage rather than progressing on to other elements of the resuscitation programme. Oxygen supplementation is used at this stage and is the most vital 'drug' of the whole resuscitation programme. Remember that the whole purpose of opening up an airway and getting some ventilation is to provide oxygen to the brain and vital organs. It is therefore important to maximise the inhaled oxygen concentration to provide as much oxygen as possible to these structures.

Circulation

Once airway and breathing have been cured, assessment of circulation and therefore perfusion of the vital organs needs to be assessed. This can be determined, not only by level of consciousness in a global way, but more specifically by heart rate, pulse, volume and presence of pulse in certain parts of the anatomy, as well as capillary refilling time, and obviously blood pressure if this can be assessed. The level of shock can be graded from 1–4. Grade 1 is determined by a 750 mL blood loss where the respiratory rate is less than 20 and the pulse rate less than 100. Grade 2 is when less than 1500 mL of blood has been lost, the respiratory rate is less than 30 and the pulse rate above 100 but less than 120. Grade 3 is when blood pressure starts to fall and this is when more than 1500 mL of volume has been lost, the respiratory rate rises to between 30 and 40 respirations a minute and the pulse rate rises to above 120. In the more severe cases of Grade 4 there is more than 2 L of blood loss, the respiratory rate rises above 40 and the pulse rate above 140. If the systolic blood pressure falls below 90 mmHg then often the radial pulse is no longer palpable and this can be a guide that shock is imminent and that an intravenous line needs to be set up and fluids started. Likewise, the presence of an open wound should be enough evidence for an i.v. line to be set up and 250 mL of saline started immediately.

The most common cause of shock is haemorrhagic shock as in significant bleeding, either externally or internally, and the therapist needs to be aware of injuries to the spleen, liver or kidney that may cause rapid loss of blood volume. Physical signs of suspected intra-abdominal haemorrhage include obvious bruising, significant abdominal pain and tenderness with guarding, rebound tenderness within the abdomen and evidence of fractured ribs. External haemorrhage is more obvious and should be treated with splinting, pressure and elevation. Throughout this element of resuscitation the circulation status needs to be constantly reassessed by pulse and blood pressure measurement.

Cervical spine

Once **A**, **B** and **C** have been controlled, it is important then to assess the cervical spine. This is easier if the player is conscious; however, if they remain unconscious one should assume a serious neck injury until proven otherwise. If the injury is witnessed and a cervical spine injury is suspected then it should be managed as a cervical spine injury and assessed appropriately even if the patient is asymptomatic initially.

If a cervical spine injury is suspected, then a collar and spinal board immobilisation needs to be performed. There is no room for compromise even if a player insists that his neck feels fine. If you, as a therapist, have a suspicion that you cannot totally exclude one, then you need to err on the side of caution until a cervical spine injury has been cleared. Again, emergency pitch-side courses are recommended to gain experience but in essence, the absence of spine tenderness, the absence of any cervical spine pain, the absence of any upper or lower limb neurological symptoms or signs and the full pain-free active range of movement of the cervical spine by the patient without any discomfort or block may suggest that there is no cervical spine injury in the player. If, however, some of these symptoms are present, it is important at this stage to immobilise the spine with a cervical collar and spinal board application. If the therapist has any doubt as to whether a cervical spine injury is present then it is prudent to err on the side of caution and immobilise the spine, even if the player insists he feels fine. The player should then be only deemed clear of cervical spine injuries when radiological evidence or further in-depth assessment has taken place.

Disability

This category covers several aspects of assessing the player's status. The level of pain needs to be assessed both in site, intensity and character. Severe pain can impair proper assessment of a player and judicious use of analgesics, including morphine and cyclizine antiemetic, would be appropriate.

The level of mental awareness and cognitive function needs to be assessed and this recorded, together with the time, as any deterioration over a period of time could be significant and very important in helping management. Glasgow coma scales, or the simple AVPU assessment, are important. Neurological assessment, including pupil examination and assessment of the myotomes and dermatomes, needs to be performed and in a situation of concussion some cognitive function questions need to be asked. In several sports where concussion is more frequent, such as horse racing, rugby union and league and Aussie Rules, a series of Maddocks questions have been devised to give the therapist a way of assessing cognitive function on the pitch. These include the following questions which can be modified for different sports:

1. Where are you?
2. Who are you playing?
3. Who is your opposite number?
4. What half are we in?
5. How far into that half?
6. Who scored last?
7. Who did we play last week?
8. Did we win or lose?

If the player gets more than one question wrong, then he should be deemed as cognitively impaired and should be removed from the field of play for further assessment.

Once the above has been assessed, then further assessment of the musculoskeletal system such as the chest wall, the pelvis and the limbs as well as the head and facial bones should be performed.

Exposure and environment

It is important at this stage, when waiting for further assistance, for the player to be protected from exposure to the extremes of temperature, be it hot or cold, as the effect of the environment can have a deleterious effect on the status of the player.

Secondary

Finally, further information needs to be gleamed from the patient before transfer to hospital, such as allergies, medication, past medical history, time of last meal or drink and the events of the injury including drugs given (AMPLE) need to be recorded, together with any readings and assessment of neurological status before transfer to hospital.

Concussion

Concussion is a topic that can be poorly covered at undergraduate level. It falls into a grey zone between normal brain function and head injuries that are seen following severe trauma such as road traffic accidents. It is not uncommon in team sports or collision sports and the therapist needs to be aware of concussion and its management.[6]

Concussion is defined as a complex pathophysiological complex affecting the brain, induced by traumatic biomechanical forces. It can be caused by a direct blow to the head or a blow elsewhere to the body with an impulsive force transmitted to the head. It results in rapid onset of short-lived impairment of neurological function that resolves spontaneously. It may result in neuropathological changes but the acute clinical symptoms largely reflect a functional disturbance rather than anything structural within the brain, and, therefore, concussion is typically associated with grossly normal structural neural imaging such as an MRI scan. The injury results in a spectrum of clinical syndromes that may or may not involve loss of consciousness. More than 90% of concussions are mild and only result in transient confusion.

There are some learning points and myths that the therapist needs to be aware of. Players may not be aware that they have suffered a concussion and are an unreliable source of information of how many previous concussions they have had. Likewise, team mates and coaches are also an unreliable source of information.

You do not have to be knocked out, lose consciousness or have post-traumatic amnesia to be concussed. These play no value in determining the prognosis or severity of the head injury.

- *Myth 1* – Once you have had a concussion you are more likely to have another one in the season.

This is false. The rate of concussion reflects the hours of rugby played and is not related to whether a player has had a concussion in the past or not. Obviously the more you play the more likely you are to have a concussion but this has no correlation to previous injury.

- *Myth 2* – If you play on with a concussion you are more likely to get further brain damage.

This is almost true. If you play on with concussion your insight and ability to assess risk is impaired so you start playing more dangerously and possibly recklessly and are more likely to injure yourself and others.

- *Myth 3* – Does repeated concussion result in cumulative brain damage?

There is evidence that chronic traumatic encephalopathy or punch-drunk syndrome is associated with a genetic predisposition, the epsilon for allele of the apolipoprotein E gene. This is found in 20% of the population and may be associated with a late onset of Alzheimer's condition. There is very little evidence or research examining the effect of repeated concussion in humans although animal studies do show there is no evidence of permanent brain damage after repeated head injury. It is felt, therefore, that those humans who carry this gene may be at increased risk of delayed onset encephalopathy if exposed to repeated head trauma. However, this is yet to be confirmed.

- *Myth 4* – Does the second impact syndrome exist?

Second impact syndrome is the catastrophic consequences resulting from a second concussive blow to a player before he is fully recovered from the symptoms of a previous concussion. These cases are often highlighted in the press and can result in collapse and death of an athlete. It is believed to be the result of loss of cerebral autoregulation causing cerebral oedema and mortality although a recent review of all the papers concludes that there is lack of evidence that cerebral oedema occurs. Despite this lack of evidence, it is important to be aware of this syndrome and as a therapist you need to be absolutely sure that all symptoms and signs of concussion are absent and that the proper protocol has been followed before a player can return to sport.

Symptoms of concussion

These can be very mild and include the following: headache, dizziness, nausea, double vision, blurred vision, unsteadiness or loss of balance, confusion, lack of awareness of details of the match, a feeling of being stunned or dazed, seeing stars or flashing lights and ringing in the ears. Signs of concussion include impaired conscious state but not necessarily loss of consciousness, poor coordination and balance, unsteady gait, slow to answer questions, easily distracted with poor concentration, unusual emotions and behaviour, feeling of nausea and vomiting, a vacant stare and glassy-eyed, slurred speech, personality changes and double vision with blurred vision.

 Pitch-side assessment

If a player has sustained a head injury, then normal emergency pitch-side protocols need to be followed such as completing the Sport Concussion Assessment Tool or SCAT (Fig. 5.1). However, as part of this, the neurological and cognitive function of the patient needs to be assessed and, as mentioned above, Maddocks questions need to be answered. If there is doubt then further assessment of the cognitive function can be made through simple question/answer procedures such as the 100 minus 7s, the months of the year backwards and the 5-item recall test. A full neurological examination is preferable but an assessment of the neck, skull, the eyes in terms of nystagmus, diplopia and field of vision, the limbs in terms of finger/nose testing, outstretched drift and power and coordination in terms of modified Romberg's test made all need to be.

If there is any doubt in any of the assessment then the player needs to be removed from the field of play and observed quietly at the edge of the pitch whilst being repeatedly assessed.

Injury management: the first 24 h

What you do to a player and how you manage his injury within the first 24 h can have dramatic affects on the duration of the injury and the long-term health of that player. Spending time to minimise the extent of the injury and maximise the healing capacity of the injury can have massive time saving benefits both for the therapist and the player and respecting this critical period is important to further management. Within the first 24 h, two important processes occur.

Haemostasis

Immediately following injury there is vasodilation followed by vasoconstriction resulting in the formation of a platelet plug coagulation and a fibrous matrix. Minimising the vasodilation and the resultant bleeding and swelling and the pressure increase that causes pain, tenderness and impaired healing is essential. This needs to be started as soon as possible and the blood needs to be encouraged to be reabsorbed into the lymphatics to be removed from the site of the injury. Within hours of injury, there is leukocyte recruitment with macrophages and neutrophils as part of the inflammatory process. This process is important for removal of debris, protection against infection and instigation of the early stages of the healing process. However, if this is excessive, then sometimes this effect can be counterproductive and can slow new tissue formation. It is important, therefore, to minimise these effects and facilitate the systems within the body of healing. Further damage to tissue structures and secondary hypoxic injury need to be avoided and this is best summarised by the letters PRICED.

*P*rotect

It is important to protect the area of the body that has been injured, to prevent any excessive movement, to prevent others from aggravating the injury and to allow the healing process to be instigated. Immobilisation is essential for certain injuries such as acute fractures and some stress fractures such as navicular fractures. Likewise, severe soft tissue injuries may need to be immobilised for 48 h to limit pain and swelling. This can be provided through crutches, braces, splints, thermoplastic materials and plaster casts.

This Tool represents a standardised method of evaluating people after concussion in sport. This Tool has been produced as part of the Summary and Agreement Statement of the Second International Symposium on Concussion in Sport, Prague 2004

Sport concussion is defined as a complex pathophysiological process affecting the brain, induced by traumatic biomechanical forces. Several common features that incorporate clinical, pathological and biomechanical injury constructs that may be utilised in defining the nature of a concussive head injury include:

1. Concussion may be caused either by a direct blow to the head, face, neck or elsewhere on the body with an 'impulsive' force transmitted to the head.
2. Concussion typically results in the rapid onset of short-lived impairment of neurological function that resolves spontaneously.
3. Consussion may result in neuropathological changes but the acute clinical symptoms largely reflect a functional disturbance rather than structural injury.
4. Concussion results in a graded set of clinical syndromes that may or may not involve loss of consciousness. Resolution of the clinical and cognitive symptoms typically follows a sequential course.
6. Concussion is typically associated with grossly normal structural neuroimaging studies.

Post Concussion Symptoms

Ask the athlete to score themselves based on how they feel now. It is recognised that a low score may be normal for some athletes, but clinical judgement should be exercised to determine if a change in symptoms has occurred following the suspected concussion event.

It should be recognised that the reporting of symptoms may not be entirely reliable. This may be due to the effects of a concussion or because the athlete's passionate desire to return to competition outweighs their natural inclination to give an honest response.

If possible, ask someone who knows the athlete well about changes in affect, personality, behaviour, etc.

Remember, concussion should be suspected in the presence of ANY ONE or more of the following:
- Symptoms (such as headache), or
- Signs (such as loss of consciousness), or
- Memory problems

Any athlete with a suspected concussion should be monitored for deterioration (ie., should not be left alone) and should not drive a motor vehicle.

For more information see the 'Summary and Agreement Statement of the Second International Symposium on Concussion in Sport' in the April, 2005 edition of the *Clinical Journal of Sport Medicine* (Vol 15), *British Journal of Sports Medicine* (Vol 39), *Neurosurgery* (Vol 59) and *The Physician and Sportsmedicine* (Vol 33). This tool may be copied for distribution to teams, groups and organizations. ©2005 Concession in Sport Group

  魔*IIHF*

The SCAT Card
(Sport Concussion Assessment Tool)
Athlete information

What is a concussion? A concussion is a disturbance in the function of the brain caused by a direct or indirect force to the head. It results in a variety of symptoms (like those listed below) and may, or may not, involve memory problems or loss of conciousness.

How do you feel? You should score yourself on the following symptoms, based on how you feel now.

Post Concussion Symptom Scale	None		Moderate			Severe	
Headache	0	1	2	3	4	5	6
'Pressure in head'	0	1	2	3	4	5	6
Neck pain	0	1	2	3	4	5	6
Balance problems or dizzy	0	1	2	3	4	5	6
Nausea or vomiting	0	1	2	3	4	5	6
Vision problems	0	1	2	3	4	5	6
Hearing problems/ringing	0	1	2	3	4	5	6
'Don't feel right'	0	1	2	3	4	5	6
Feeling 'dinged' or 'dazed'	0	1	2	3	4	5	6
Confusion	0	1	2	3	4	5	6
Feeling slowed down	0	1	2	3	4	5	6
Feeling like 'in a fog'	0	1	2	3	4	5	6
Drowsiness	0	1	2	3	4	5	6
Fatigue or low energy	0	1	2	3	4	5	6
More emotional than usual	0	1	2	3	4	5	6
Irritability	0	1	2	3	4	5	6
Difficulty concentrating	0	1	2	3	4	5	6
Difficulty remembering	0	1	2	3	4	5	6

(Follow up symptoms only)

	None		Moderate			Severe	
Sadness	0	1	2	3	4	5	6
Nervous or anxious	0	1	2	3	4	5	6
Trouble falling asleep	0	1	2	3	4	5	6
Sleeping more than usual	0	1	2	3	4	5	6
Sensitivity to light	0	1	2	3	4	5	6
Sensitivity to noise	0	1	2	3	4	5	6
Other: _____	0	1	2	3	4	5	6

What should I do?
Any athlete suspected of having a concussion should be removed from play, and then seek medical evaluation.

Signs to watch for:
Problems could arise over the first 24–48 h. You should not be left alone and must go to a hospital at once if you:
- Have a headache that gets worse
- Are very drowsy or can't be awakened (woken up)
- Can't recognise people or places
- Have repeated vomiting
- Behave unusually or seem confused; are very irritable
- Have seizures (arms and legs jerk uncontrollably)
- Have weak or numb arms or legs
- Are unsteady on your feet; have slurred speech
Remember, it is better to be safe. Consult your doctor after a suspected concussion.

What can I expect?
Concussion typically results in the rapid onset of short-lived impairment that resolves spontaneously over time. You can expect that you will be told to rest until you are fully recovered (that means resting your body and your mind). Then, your doctor will likely advise that you go through a gradual increase in exercise over several days (or longer) before returning to sport.

Figure 5.1 (A,B) Sport Concussion Assessment Tool (SCAT) cards.[7]

FIFA $\bigcirc\bigcirc\bigcirc$ *IIHF*

The SCAT Card
(Sport Concussion Assessment Tool)
Medical Evaluation

Name: _____ Date: _____

Sport/Team: _____ Mouth guard? Y N

1) SIGNS
Was there loss of consciousness or unresponsiveness? Y N
Was there seizure or convulsive activity? Y N
Was there a balance problem/unsteadiness? Y N

2) MEMORY
Modified Maddocks questions (check correct)

At what venue are we? __ ; Which half is it? __ ; Who scored last? __;

What team did we play last? __ ; Did we win last game? __?

3) SYMPTOM SCORE
Total number of positive symptoms
(from reverse side of the card) = _____

4) COGNITIVE ASSESSMENT

5 word recall   Immediate   Delayed
                      (Examples)   (after concentration
                                                       tasks)

Word 1 _____   cat   _____   _____
Word 2 _____   pen   _____   _____
Word 3 _____   shoe   _____   _____
Word 4 _____   book   _____   _____
Word 5 _____   car   _____   _____

Months in reverse order:
Jun-May-April-Mar-Feb-Jan-Dec-Nov-Oct-Sep-Aug-Jul
(circle incorrect)   *or*

Digits backwards (check correct)
5-2-8-   3-9-1   _____
6-2-9-4   4-3-7-1   _____
8-3-2-7-9   1-4-9-3-6   _____
7-3-9-1-4-2   5-1-8-4-6-8 _____
            Ask delayed 5-word recall

5) NEUROLOGICAL SCREENING
                          Pass   Fail
Speech   _____   _____
Eye motion and pupils   _____   _____
Pronator drift   _____   _____
Gait assessment   _____   _____

*Any neurologic screening abnormality necessitates formal
neurologic or hospital assessment*

6) RETURN TO PLAY
Athletes should not be returned to play the same day of injury.
When returning athletes to play, they should follow a stepwise
symptom-limited programme, with stages of progression. For
example:
  1. Rest until asymptomatic (physical and mental rest)
  2. Light aerobic exercise (e.g. stationary cycle)
  3. Sport-specific exercise
  4. Non-contact training drills (start light resistance training)
  5. Full contact training after medical clearance
  6. Return to competition (game play)

There should be approximately 24 hours (or longer) for each
stage and the athlete should return to stage 1 if symptoms recur.
Resistance training should only be added in the later stages.
Medical clearance should be given before return to play.

Instructions:
This side of the card is for the use of medical
doctors, physiotherapists or athletic therapists.
In order to maximise the information gathered
from the card, it is strongly suggested that all
athletes participating in contact sports
complete a baseline evaluation prior to the
beginning of their competetive season. This
card is a suggested guide only for sports
concussion and is not meant to assess more
severe forms of brain injury. **Please give a
COPY of this card to the athlete for their
information and to guide follow-up
assessment.**

Signs:
Assess for each of these items and circle
Y (yes) or N (no).

Memory: If needed, questions can be
modified to make them specific to the sport
(e.g. 'period' versus'half').

Cognitive assessment:
Select any 5 words (an example is given).
Avoid choosing related words such as 'dark'
and 'moon' which can be recalled by means of
word association. Read each word at a rate of
one word per second. The athlete should not
be informed of the delayed testing of memory
(to be done after the reverse months and/or
digits). Choose a difficult set of words each
time you perform a follow-up exam with
the same candidate.
Ask the athlete to recite the months of the
year in reverse order, starting with a random
month. Do not start with December or
January. Circle any months not recited in the
correct sequence.
For digits backwards, if correct, go to the
next string length. If incorrect, read trial 2.
Stop after incorrect on both trials.

Neurologic screening:
Trained medical personnel must administer
this examination. These individuals might
include medical doctors, physiotherapists or
athletic therapists. Speech should be
assessed for fluency and lack of slurring. Eye
motion should reveal no doploia in any of the
4 planes of movement (vertical, horizontal and
both diagonal planes). The pronator drift is
performed by asking the patient to hold both
arms in front of them, palms up, with eyes
closed. A positive test is pronating the forearm,
dropping the arm, or drift away from midline.
For gait assessment, ask the patient to
walk away from you, turn and walk back.

Return to play:
A structured, graded exertion protocol should
be developed; individualised on the basis of
sport, age and the concussion history of the
athlete. Exercise or training should be
commenced only after the athlete is clearly
asymptomatic with physical and cognitive rest.
Final decision for clearance to return to
competition should ideally be made by a
medical doctor.

For more information see the 'Summary and
Agreement Statement of the Second
International Symposium on Concussion in
Sport' in the April 2005 *Clinical Journal of
Sport Medicine* (Vol 15), *British Journal of
Sports Medicine* (Vol 39), *Neurosurgery*
(Vol 59) and the *Physician and
Sportsmedicine* (Vol 33). ©2005 Concession
in Sport Group

Figure 5.1, cont'd

*R*est

Similar to protection, it is important that the athlete rests the area injured so as to decrease bleeding and swelling. The use of slings or crutches is important in this to remind the player that they need to treat their limb with respect.

*I*ce

The principal behind using ice therapy is to provide vasoconstriction and analgesia. Although there is no high quality evidence for how this should be applied, it is generally accepted that applying ice for 15 min every 1–2 h initially and then gradually reducing the frequency over the next 24 h is common practice. Ice should not be applied to areas of poor circulation and the player needs to be advised of the risk of skin burns and nerve damage with prolonged ice application. The use of crushed ice in a moist bag, ice immersion in a bucket or a bath are the most common forms of this application.

*C*ompression

Compression of an injured area reduces bleeding and minimises swelling and the application of ice should not delay any compression. Evidence suggests that it is not used enough even though it plays a major role in reducing oedema around an injury. Compression should start just distal to the site of the bleeding or injury and should extend 6 inches proximal to the injury. Compression should be progressive and encourage any fluid to move in a cardiac direction. Compression has been shown to be more effective than ice, elevation or rest in reducing oedema and swelling around an injury.

*E*levation

This reduces oedema and accumulation of interstitial fluid around an injury and again is underused. The use of a sling or resting an upper limb on a tower of pillows on the arm of a chair whilst sitting in a chair has been found useful. Also, elevation of a lower limb on a chair or pillows has been shown to be of benefit, as opposed to standing for prolonged periods of time where a dependant foot may become more swollen.

*D*rugs

Historically, early use of antiinflammatories has been beneficial. As mentioned above, it is important that some form of inflammatory process is allowed to occur and the routine use of antiinflammatories in all injuries is now not being recommended. It is important that control of pain with simple analgesics is advised and the use of paracetamol or some codeine-related drugs is a good first-line treatment; however antiinflammatories within the first 24 h may be of limited benefit.

Injury management: after 24 h

There are a variety of treatment modalities that have beneficial effects on a variety of injuries. Not all these treatment regimes apply to every injury; however, the modalities that are available are outlined below with some of their benefits highlighted.

Mobilisation

After an initial period of immobilisation, some degree of movement of the tissues has benefits. It prevents stiffness, allows articular cartilage nourishment and maintains some degree of muscle strength. Free restraint movement, however, may be more than the delicate healing tissues can tolerate and therefore limited movement within a brace or within taping may be advised. Early mobilisation of a joint such as an ankle sprain decreases the pain and swelling and improves functional outcomes compared to those that are left in a cast for prolonged periods of time. Movement may be facilitated by continuous passive motion. This benefits in a similar way by encouraging articular cartilage nutrition and reducing joint stiffness and is useful in the early stages of muscular injuries.

Hot and cold therapy

The use of cryotherapy in the acute stages as part of PRICED has been mentioned above. Ice massage has been used in specific local, superficial conditions such as a tendinopathy where a cube of ice has been massaged in a circular fashion over a superficial tendon for 5–10 min. This gives an analgesic effect by decreasing motor and sensory nerve conduction velocity.

Heat therapy may contribute to improved treatment of soft tissue injuries but should not be used within the first 48 h. The use of heat treatment and hot towels has been used for many years in easing muscle spasm around an injury and to facilitate rehabilitation. The use of contrast baths of alternating hot and cold is felt to decrease swelling by creating an alternating mechanical force.

Therapeutic modalities

A large variety of electrotherapeutic modalities have been used over the years, some with very little evidence but a summary of their effects is as follows.

Ultrasound

This is meant to increase local blood flow, settle the metabolism and reduce pain through the thermal effect of ultrasound; however, clinical trials showing its efficacy have been poorly designed and there is little evidence to support ultrasound treatment on soft tissue injuries. Low intensity pulsed ultrasound has been, however, shown to be successful in acute fractures as well as those showing delayed or non-union. This is applied for 20 min/day in contrast to traditional ultrasound, which lasts for no more than 5 min. The effect of low intensity pulse ultrasound has been shown to reduce healing time and thus return to sport time and is increasingly used in rehabilitation.

TENS

Transcutaneous electrical nerve stimulation (TENS) provides pain relief through a direct current applied across the skin. High frequency TENS can provide good pain relief initially but sometimes patients become tolerant. After providing pain relief this allows the patient to mobilise the joint or injured area and facilitate rehabilitation. A low frequency TENS acts like an acupuncture-like analgesic and is more useful on trigger points or muscle spasms.

Interferential stimulation

This is a form of TENS in which two alternating currents are simultaneously applied to the skin, thus stimulating the muscle in a similar manner to normal muscle contraction. It acts as pain relief and reduces oedema and swelling as well as stimulating muscle and increasing cell activity.

Neuromuscular stimulators

These are primarily used to maintain strength and flexibility and reduce atrophy during the healing process. They are similar to a TENS machine; however, they have an on/off button which allows muscles to contract and then to relax before the next contraction. The theory is that they will provide muscle contraction under stimulation and therefore reduce atrophy, thus speeding up rehabilitation. There is little research to prove this although it is commonly used in practice.

Laser treatment

Laser stands for 'light amplification by stimulated emission of radiation' and can be high powered lasers used in industry and low or middle powered lasers, known as coal lasers, used in the treatment of soft tissue injuries. They are meant to reduce pain, swelling and inflammation and provide muscle stimulation but there is little evidence that they help in musculoskeletal pain. However, there is some evidence to suggest that low level lasers may be effective in treating subacute tendinopathies.

Extra corporeal shockwave therapy

ESWT has been used in the treatment of tendinopathies and fracture non-unions. Research papers have shown conflicting results of the effectiveness of this treatment in these two conditions, although it is commonly used in the treatment of tendinopathy. More specifically, however, it has been used in the treatment of calcific tendinopathy, especially in the supraspinatus tendon, Achilles and patella tendon. It can be a painful procedure but still has a role to play in the management of tendon injuries.

Acupuncture and dry needling

There are many subtypes of acupuncture ranging from the ancient Chinese classical method to the more modern adapted use of acupuncture either over acupuncture points or over areas of muscle tension and spasm. Its exact mechanism of action is uncertain although the autonomic nervous system may play an important role in addition to the release of endorphins. Both of these have a function in the pain pathways as well as the reduction of muscle spasm and trigger point activity.

An extension from acupuncture is dry needling, both of tendon injuries and over the periosteum in bony bruising. The theory behind this stems from the assumption that the resultant local bleeding that occurs as a result of dry needling brings with it some healing factors or growth factors that may promote faster healing. The use of dry needling in tendinopathies has been used extensively and at times has superseded the injections of steroids to equal effect.

An extension of this argument has resulted in the injections of autologous blood in the understanding that by actually injecting small amounts of blood into the tendons you are actually encouraging more of the effect of dry needling and this has been performed under ultrasound control into various tendons with encouraging results.

Manual therapy

The details of manual therapy are beyond the scope of this book; however, suffice to say that joints, muscles and neural structures can be treated by manual therapy with beneficial effect. Joint mobilisation aims to restore range of movement in a previously stiff or painful joint and is aimed at working within the physiological joint range to mimic normal function and restore, not only normal range of movement, but accessory movement patterns.

Joint manipulation is the use of sudden movements or thrusts of small amplitude performed at high speed at the end of range of joint movement. These are movements that the patient is unable to reproduce themselves and are aimed at increasing the range of movement within a joint. These actions are confined to those therapists with extra training and are often used at intervertebral joints to increase the range of movement.

Muscle soft tissue therapy, or massage therapy, is used extensively to reduce thickened or tight connective tissue, to release myofascial trigger points that inhibit muscle contraction or cause pain and are used to reduce muscle tone and tension. There are various techniques including digital pressure and sustained myofascial tension but also soft and deep tissue massage, cupping and fascial massage, all of which have beneficial effects in reducing pain, improving neuromuscular control, improving range of movement and removing inhibitory triggers that reduce power, endurance and muscle activity.

Drug therapy

As mentioned above, the use of non-steroidal antiinflammatory drugs is wide among sporting injuries. They were first used on the assumption that excessive inflammation was a negative thing and that this needed to be stopped. Unfortunately, there is very little evidence of their benefit and their use is reducing in sporting injuries. Their benefit may have been perceived through their analgesic effect and anti-pyretic effect rather than their antiinflammatory effect. Their role may have some benefit in obvious inflammatory disorders such as inflammatory arthritis, bursitis and enthesopathies that may be associated with rheumatological conditions. However, in most soft tissue injuries, use of simple analgesics, such as paracetamol, may be equally as good. If one is prescribing an antiinflammatory, one has to make a conscious decision as to what inflammatory condition you are treating and how long you plan to treat that condition for. Prescriptions for prolonged courses of antiinflammatories have often resulted in unwanted side-effects; mainly gastrointestinal dyspepsia and have given antiinflammatories a bad name. Certainly, after 2 weeks of antiinflammatories, the benefit may be purely analgesic rather than antiinflammatory. It is therefore recommended that if you are prescribing antiinflammatories you do so purely for an inflammatory condition and confine the treatment to 5–10 days' duration. This obviously does not include rheumatological conditions which often need prolonged courses of antiinflammatories under the care of a consultant rheumatologist.

Corticosteroids

The use of corticosteroids is a highly controversial issue. They can be administered by local injection, by oral ingestion or by iontophoresis. Their aim is to reduce pain and inflammation so that a productive rehabilitation programme can commence and they should be considered as a 'helping hand' up the treatment ladder to provide some relief while other issues are addressed.

Local corticosteroid injections have been used for many years in the treatment of bursitis, tendinopathy, arthritis and synovitis. The side-effects of steroids include the local side-effects of skin atrophy and skin discoloration as well as possible local infection and the systemic effects of loss of blood pressure and diabetic control, flushing and hormonal imbalance. It must be emphasised that corticosteroids inhibit collagen synthesis and tissue repair and these effects seem to be dose related. Likewise, the injection of corticosteroids into weight-bearing joints may have a deleterious effect on the articular cartilage and should be limited in number.

Evidence for corticosteroid injection benefit is limited. There is no evidence but anecdotally it does help. Like non-steroidal antiinflammatory drugs, its use should really be confined to those conditions that are purely inflammatory such as bursitis or inflammatory arthritis and the number of injections to any one site should be restricted. Successive injections should not be performed more frequently than 3–4-weekly.

The role of corticosteroids in tendinopathy is more contentious. Inaccurate injections of steroids into the tendon itself have an increased role in tendon rupture and the medico–legal consequences that go with this. It is therefore advised that corticosteroid injections around tendons should be performed accurately with ultrasound control. However, their role is still contentious as biopsies of tendinopathies have failed to show any evidence of acute inflammation. It is because of this that dry needling and subsequent use of autologous blood has superseded corticosteroid injections.

Oral corticosteroids are very rarely used in the sports injury field, mainly because they are banned by the IOC. However, they may have a beneficial effect in acute cervical disc radiculopathy, osteitis pubis or chronic tendinopathies. A limited course of oral prednisolone, 25–30 mg/day for 5 days, may be beneficial with minimal detrimental effects; however, possible complications always include avascular necrosis of the femoral head.

Iontophoresis is the administration of topical steroids through the skin for superficial bursitis or tendinopathies. They seem to give rapid onset analgesic effects and can facilitate rehabilitation although there is little research evidence to prove this.

Tendinopathy

Chronic tendinopathy is a difficult problem to treat and several drugs have been used in its management. Steroids, as mentioned above, and other drugs have been used in this field with varying degrees of success.

Sclerosant treatment

Ultrasound scanning of chronic tendinopathies has shown the presence of neovascularisation. The presence of this seems to be proportional to the degree of pain and severity of the condition although this statement is still contentious. It is therefore felt that obliterating these endovascular vessels can play a role in assisting with chronic pain and tendinopathy. The use of sclerosant therapy, such as polidocanol which acts as an irritant to the vessels, has been shown to be of benefit. It is injected under ultrasound control, not into the tendon but into the tendon area, and has been shown to significantly reduce pain and allow the patient to return to pain-free tendon loading activity.

Glyceryl trinitrate

This has been used also as a vasodilator and a stimulant of collagen synthesis. Its topical use over superficial tendons such as supraspinatus and Achilles tendon shows a beneficial effect over a 6-month period when used with other conventional Achilles rehabilitation programmes.

Aprotinin

This is a collagen inhibitor which is not available in the UK under licence but has been used in other countries in the form of injection therapy for tendinopathy in the hope that this will regenerate collagen formation. Results are encouraging but it is in the early stages and the jury is still out on its effectiveness.

Take home points

- Be aware of the useful acronyms in injury management: DR ABCDES in pitch-side care, and PRICED in the first 24 h of an injury.
- Name the different types of acute and overuse injuries for different parts of the body.
- What are the signs and symptoms of concussion?

CLINICAL CASE

You are presented with a 20-year-old elite Taekwondo athlete who has come to see you for advice.

Some 3 weeks ago he was competing in a competition when he was kicked on the point of his chin. He was knocked out for 20 s and was helped off the competition mat, recovered very quickly on the side and there were no residual symptoms of nausea, headache or visual upset. He felt well but he was eliminated from the competition and he did not compete further.

On returning home he continued to train and felt well without any sequelae. Four days prior to seeing you he was again involved in a qualifying competition and was kicked on the side of the head and again was knocked out. This was only the second time he had ever been knocked out. He apparently lost consciousness for almost 45 seconds and again was eliminated from the competition, helped off the competitive surface and was assessed in the medical tent. At that time he remembers having a headache, and feeling dizzy and slightly nauseous, which persisted for 3 h. He has come home and since then has not trained or performed any exercise and no longer has any nausea, vomiting, headache, dizziness or visual upset, but admits to feeling irritable, has not slept well since he has returned, and although he cannot put his finger exactly on it, says he does not feel 100%.

He is due to fly out to Morocco the following day for a final Olympic qualifying competition in 10 days time. This will be the last opportunity he has to qualify for the Olympics, which has been his target for the last 4 years. He has not been able to compete in the last two Olympics, the first because he had broken his leg and the second because he had glandular fever. There is no team doctor, although there will be a physiotherapist and an event doctor at the competition in Morocco.

On examination he appears well and was alert and talked coherently. He had no restriction of his range of movement of his neck and had no bony abnormality or tenderness over his chin, cheek or facial bones. Full examination of his central and peripheral nervous system was normal, including fundoscopy. Examination of his pupils which were equally reactive to light, his power, tone reflexes and sensation were all normal, as was his coordination. Cognitively he was orientated in time and place, and successfully recalled a 5-item recall at 1, 3, 5 and 10 min. He completed the 100 −7s test correctly as well as the months of the year backwards test correctly. Unfortunately he has no previous cognitive baseline test to which you can compare.

How would you advise him regarding his present diagnosis, his management and whether he should compete, or indeed travel to Morocco?

This Taekwondo athlete is still suffering from a complex concussion. It appears from the first injury, 3 weeks before you saw him, that although he was knocked out he was not concussed. He had no symptoms of concussion at the time of the injury, and was able to exercise without symptoms following this. The second injury, 4 days prior to the consultation, however, was different. He again was knocked out and lost consciousness, although this is not necessarily a feature of concussion. He did, however, have symptoms of concussion including a headache, dizziness and nausea for 3 h after the event. Although those symptoms had subsided, he was having persistent symptoms of irritability, sleep disturbance and not feeling 100%, 4 days later. This represents a complex concussion, one that needs to be monitored before returning to any form of exercise.

Examination both of his cognitive function and neurological system was perfectly normal, and therefore it is highly unlikely that he had any underlying neurological dysfunction. It is difficult to monitor his recovery as he plans to fly to Morocco for this final qualifying competition. There is no contraindication to him flying, however, it is important for him to understand that his re-grading back into activity should be monitored closely by his medical staff, and he understands the importance of not competing until he has had a significant period of being symptom-free and re-grading with exercise also without symptoms.

Advice given to him is that he is to refrain from any form of exercise until he is free of all his symptoms for 48 hours, then he can re-grade over a period of time as follows:

- Day 1: 20 min light cycling only
- Day 2: 20–30 min 50–60% running only
- Day 3. More intensive training session of 1 h duration but not involving contact
- Day 4. Be cleared as fit for contact by medical personnel at the medical department in Morocco
- Day 5. Fit for contact training.

It is important that he not only follows these rules of re-grading but remains symptom-free during these forms of exercise and for the 24 h afterwards. If he develops any symptoms then he must refrain from all activity for 24 h and then restart the re-grading programme at one step below that which his symptoms started.

In an ideal world, he would be given the all clear by a consultant neurologist, who may want to arrange brain imaging, although by definition this will be normal if he has concussion. Also it would be preferred if you could compare a cognitive baseline test with a similar test at day 4, either a join-the-dots test, or a symbol test or ideally a computer-generated Cogsport test. However, none of these are available to him as there is no baseline with which to compare.

The instructions outlined above should be written down and given to him as well as to any doctor who will be looking after his care while abroad. He was informed that the chances of him being fit to compete were only 50/50 and that it was vitally important that he was entirely symptom-free throughout his re-grading and when returning to contact training before being cleared to compete.

REFERENCES

1. Garrett WE Jr. Muscle strain injuries. Am J Sports Med 1996; 24(Suppl 6):S2–S8.
2. Brukner P, Bennell K, Matheson G. Stress fractures. Melbourne: Blackwell Scientific; 1999.
3. Heckman JD, Ryaby JP, McCabe J, et al. Acceleration of tibial fracture-healing by non-invasive, low-intensity pulsed ultrasound. J Bone Joint Surg Am 1994; 76(1):26–34.
4. Jozsa K. Human tendons. Champaign, IL: Human Kinetics; 1997.
5. Pitchside Immediate Trauma Care Course in association with the Faculty of Pre-Hospital Care and Resuscitation Council (UK).
6. McCrory P. CogSport. The complete concussion management system, handbook. Version 2.2. Melbourne: CogState.

7. McCrory P, Johnston K, Meeuwisse W et al. Summary and agreement statement of the 2nd International Conference on Concussion in Sport, Prague 2004. Br J Sports Med 2005; 39:196–204.

FURTHER READING

Brukner P, Kahn K. Clinical sports medicine. 3rd edn. Maidenhead: McGraw-Hill; 2006.

Chapter | 6 |

Return to sport

Returning an athlete to their sport as quickly as possible following an injury is the challenge to sports medics today. The athlete's aim is often to return to the sport as quickly as they possibly can from the injury, so it is the sports medic's job to guide them through this process, while also working to prevent a recurrence of the injury.

Consequently, a sports medic must have a clear understanding of the pathophysiology that will occur after an injury, together with an in-depth understanding of what the athlete's sport or event actually entails. This knowledge base will allow the sports medic to accurately plan a treatment and rehabilitation

© 2009 Elsevier Ltd, Inc, BV
DOI: 10.1016/B978-0-443-06813-3.00009-0

programme which takes into consideration both the physiological processes of healing which are occurring and the full physical demands of the athlete.

THE INFLAMMATORY PROCESS AND TISSUE HEALING

Once a tissue in the body is injured, it undergoes the same process each time to repair itself. The process is a very complicated, chemically mediated reaction and therefore a simplified version of this process will be discussed here.

Bleeding phase

An injury causes bleeding to occur in the injured tissue and this starts immediately after the injury has been caused. The bleeding lasts for about 8 h on average, although in vascular tissue and after significant injuries, it can continue for up to 24 h after the event.

This is an important timeframe to remember when treating the acute injury to prevent further and excessive bleeding, and therefore, the PRICE guidelines discussed earlier are vital in this early phase.

Inflammatory phase

The inflammatory phase begins just a few hours after the injury has occurred and is a vital part of the repair process. The actual peak of the inflammatory process is approximately 2–3 days after the injury, although the process will continue over the next 1–2 weeks although it will diminish over this time.

The trauma or injury causes the release of inflammatory mediators (such as mast cells and basophils) which in turn trigger a vascular and cellular response. The vascular response caused by these mediators is vasodilation and increased permeability of the cells which leads to increased blood flow and increased inflammatory exudate or fluid, which is the swelling associated with any injury.

The cellular response causes phagocytes to be released which clear up the dead or damaged tissue. In turn, these macrophages mediate the beginning of the proliferative phase by releasing chemicals at the end of their phagocytic process.

Proliferative or repair phase

The proliferative phase also begins at between 24 and 48 h, although it does not reach its peak activity levels for some 2–3 weeks. It continues thereafter but the activity diminishes over the next few weeks.

One of the types of cell that migrate to the damaged tissue due to the chemical mediators released by the macrophages are the fibroblasts. These fibroblasts are responsible for collagen synthesis and angiogenesis (new circulation formation) and it is with this collagen synthesis that the repair occurs. The collagen fibres are laid down along the lines of stress to the tissue and this is an important phase for the athlete to begin their loading, so as to ensure that the collagen fibres are aligned in the right direction.

Remodelling phase

The remodelling phase begins between 1 and 2 weeks after the injury occurs and continues for up to 1 year after the injury.

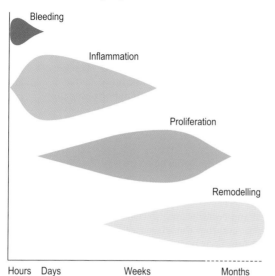

Tissue repair phases and timescale

Bleeding

Inflammation

Proliferation

Remodelling

Hours   Days   Weeks   Months

Figure 6.1 Tissue repair phases and timescale. Reproduced from *Electrotherapy on the web*, by Tim Watson, with permission (www. electrotherapy.org).

It is during this phase that the collagen matures through the maturation process and the collagen becomes stronger. As the load also increases through the tissue as the athlete returns to training and even playing, the collagen fibres align themselves more appropriately as they should be. The type I collagen that was laid down during the proliferative phase is replaced by type III collagen and the collagen or scar tissue begins to become more like the original tissue (Fig. 6.1).

FACTORS THAT DETRACT FROM HEALING

The use of antiinflammatories (NSAIDs)

Traditionally, NSAIDs have been prescribed by doctors after all injuries to try and control swelling and pain. However, numerous recent studies have shown that NSAIDs actually inhibit the release of the fibroblasts and therefore delay collagen synthesis. This leads to the scarring taking longer to occur and it is also weaker than if no NSAIDs had been given.

Therefore, other modalities such as in the PRICE guidelines should be used to control swelling and simple analgesia given if there is a need for pain control.

Alcohol after injury

Alcohol is a vasodilator and therefore causes a general increase in blood flow and limits the body's ability to form blood clots; this is especially important directly after injuries, as injuries may bleed more and for longer if athletes drink alcohol in the hours after sustaining their injury.

It is therefore very important that sports medics understand this process so that they allow the injured athlete to rest in the early stages and gradually begin loading the injured tissue when the proliferative phase begins to ensure that the collagen is laid down in the right direction and becomes as strong as possible.

THE PRINCIPLES OF REHABILITATION

A successful rehabilitation programme needs to address some key areas:

1. The programme must be devised with the healing of the tissue in mind so that a sound physiological basis for starting each different exercise is present and they can be integrated into the programme
2. The specific strengthening requirements to rehabilitate or protect the injured tissue, bearing in mind the physical demands of the activity or sport
3. Other factors such as proprioception which play a vital role for the injured tissue
4. Other associated areas which require attention to prevent the recurrence of the injury, such as core or proximal stability
5. Sport-specific aspects for the athlete, such as tackling in rugby players or the serve in tennis players, etc.
6. Discussions with technical and conditioning staff are required to ensure that overload does not occur and that the athlete will be fully prepared for when they are reintegrated into their normal training regimes
7. A plan for the gradual reintegration into full training and playing is required to ensure that the athlete does not break down as they return to the increased intensity of training and playing
8. A maintenance programme. Once athletes have returned to full training and playing, they often neglect the exercises and preventative work that had rehabilitated them. It is important that they maintain their fitness status by continuing with a maintenance programme to help protect them from recurrence.

If these factors, together with the other principles of developing goals are used, successful rehabilitation programmes can be devised, which will enable athletes to safely return to playing with the hope that recurrence is less likely.

Goal setting

Goal setting is often popular with both athletes and sports medics alike. It allows a plan to be put in place with timeframes allocated to each goal and gives the player something to aim at. However, it is important that the sports medic and athlete are realistic when they are going through this process. The goals should include both short-term and long-term goals and they should therefore go through the SMART programme below to ensure that the maximum benefit is gained from the rehabilitation programme.

Specific
• Goals should be specific to the individual and relevant to their performance. For example there is no point giving a sprinter a set time to achieve for running 800 m if they do not normally train in that way.

Measurable
• Giving the athlete exercises that can have a measured outcome is an excellent way to monitor progress and show the athlete that they are improving. It also gives a marker as to when that specific goal has been achieved so that the athlete can move onto the next one.

Achievable
• It is important that the goals are realistic to the individual athlete. It will become disheartening if they are unable to achieve any of their objectives and are not able to move along through their rehabilitation programme.

Realistic
- In a similar way to the achievable section above, there is no point asking an athlete to set a personal best or world record while they are initially recovering from an injury.

Timed
- The athlete and each goal need to have a timeframe to work to. This will give targets that the athlete can aim for, but it can also map out the whole rehabilitation process and give the athlete 'the light at the end of the tunnel'.

REHABILITATION PROGRAMMES

When writing rehabilitation programmes, it is important that the instructions are clear and that the athletes can monitor their own progress.

The template in Figure 6.2 is an example of one to use with athletes – it is easy to follow and fill in. The example includes the weights and rehabilitation exercise programme for an athlete recovering from an anterior labral repair of the shoulder, who is approximately 10 weeks postoperative.

Rehab progression records (Fig. 6.3) should be included after the description but within the programme to allow athletes to record their progress.

This programme is to be combined with a proprioceptive programme which should be done as a second session later in the day and ensures a full recovery, and is highlighted in Figure 6.4.

Return to running programme

The return to running and its progression, after an athlete has sustained an injury, has always been difficult to accurately quantify.

Figure 6.5 is a programme using an example of an athlete returning from a hamstring muscle strain. Although the example is for a hamstring injury, the running aspects and progressions can be used for any lower limb injury.

The athlete can do more than one phase in the same rehabilitation session, although it is important to gain feedback throughout the session to find out how the athlete is feeling with each phase. This is important in case they suffer pain or swelling after the session so that it is clear which aspect of the session has caused them the difficulty.

As the athlete progresses through the programme, it is important that the volume also increases so that the athlete has a functional endurance capacity before they return to full training.

Common injuries and examples of rehabilitation programmes

Knee injuries

A programme can be used for the rehabilitation of ligament and meniscal injuries in the mid stages of their recovery (without the need for weights). Figure 6.6 is an example of a programme that gives the athlete all the necessary components, with functional exercises which require a proprioceptive element to the strengthening exercises as all the exercises are in a closed kinetic chain. Figure 6.7 shows the first exercise in the programme which is VMO lunge and is a very useful exercise to include in such a rehabilitation progamme.

Name: ....

Date: ....

Definitions

- **Speed of movement:** in a second count for: – time of push, hold, return, pause i.e. 2-1-2-2 = push to count of 2 s, hold for count of 1, return to count of 2, pause for 2.
- **Range of movt:** F = full. I = inner range, M = mid-range, Iso = static hold
- **Load:** use as much load that allows you to just complete set – therefore ↑ or ↓ load as required to complete sets and reps (if you can do +3 reps on last set – ↑ load)
- Circle when weight changes

No.	Exercise	Sets	Reps/set	Load (kg)	Rest between sets	Speed of movt	Range of movt
1	Dumb-bell bench	3	8	24	30 s	1-1-1-1	F
2	Bench row	3	8	24	30 s	1-1-1-1	F
3	Front raises	3	8	10	30 s	1-1-1-1	F
4	Lateral raises	3	8	10	30 s	1-1-1-1	F
5	Cable Medial rotn @ 90° Ab/LR From high to low just turning over – quick over, slow back	3	8	2 blocks	30 s	1-1-1-1	F
6	Cable Lateral rotn @ 90° Ab From low to high, control scapula	3	8	2 blocks	30 s	1-1-1-1	F
7	Bicep Curl and Press Control scapula and no forward shoulder movt	3	8	12	30 s	1-1-1-1	F
8	Tricep dips Hands on bench, dips ensuring no forward movt of shoulders	3	12	Body weight	30 s	1-1-1-1	F

Figure 6.2 Rehabilitation programme template – an example of a programme following shoulder surgery.

	Exercise	Day 1		Day 2		Day 3		Day 4	
		Date	Load	Date	Load	Date	Load	Date	Load
1	Dumb-bell bench								
2	Bench row								
3	Front raises								
4	Lateral raises								
5	Cable medial rotation								
6	Cable medial rotation								
7	Bicep curl and press								
8	Tricep dips								

Figure 6.3 Rehab progression records.

No.	Exercise	Sets	Reps/ set	Load (kg)	Rest between sets	Speed of movt	Range of movt
1	BOSU press-ups	3	12	–	30 s	1-1-1-1	F
2	Medicine ball at wall 3 positions – full flex: 90° Ab/LR; 90° Ab + elb ext	3	20	5	30 s	–	–
3	Medial rotation catches cables high start, turn over quickly, slow control back	3	10	1–2 blocks	30 s	1-1-2-1	F
4	Medicine ball catching On bed, arm up-and-out, catch ball and flick ball up	3	10	3–5	30 s	–	–
5	Horizontal pull and catch With cables at sh level, quick pull across, slow back	3	10	2 blocks	30 s	1-1-2-1	F
6	Barbell rotations Bar above head, rotate down slowly, then back up	3	10	20	30 s	2-1-2-1	F

Figure 6.4 A shoulder proprioceptive programme.

Phase	Exercise	Intensity/ volume	End goal
1 – Acute	– Walking – Passive hamstring stretch	– Normal – Passive	– Painfree walking – 120° knee ext in neutral sitting
2 – Jog	– Light jog, with minimal acceleration/deceleration, up to 1 km	– Up to 60–70%	– Painfree jog
3 – Progressive running	– 90 metre running (straight line only) – 30 m acceleration phase – 30 m holding phase – 30 m deceleration phase	– Up to 80% in acceleration phase – 6 reps, 3 sets	– Painfree run to 80% – 3 sets completed
4 – Early acceleration deceleration	– 90 m running – Shorten the acceleration and deceleration phases – 60 m running – Shorten each phase to 20m	– Up to 90% – 6 reps, 3 sets	– Painfree to 90% – 3 sets completed – Painfree resisted knee flex in prone – Painfree full stretch
5 – Offline	– Zig-zag running over 60–80 m – start with long, slow corners – progress to gentle, over exaggerated side-steps	– Up to 60 % only – 6 reps, 3 sets	– Painfree offline – running completed
6 – Strengthening (eccentric bias)	– Hamstring strengthening programme given (no Nordics for first few days) – Ensure continuance of Core Stability programmes	– Divide prog. into 2 initially and do alternately	– Painfree completion, with full hamstring control – Maintenance of good core stability
7 – Forwards/ backwards	– Forward/backward running over 5–10 m – Gradual increase in speed and acceleration	– Build to 80% – 10 shuttles, 3 sets	– Painfree with increasing speed and acceleration achieved
8 – Standing starts	– 40–60 m run throughs – Standing starts for running progressing acceleration phase	– Up to 90% – 6 reps, 3 sets	– Painfree full run throughs to 90%
9 – Sport specific	– Integrate sport specific (ball) drills and functional movement patterns	– To 90% – Variable	– No reaction
10 – Full speed	– All above drills completed to 100% run	– 100% – Variable number of drills	– No reaction to run at full pace
11 – Contact/ resistance	– Contact drills/tackling	– 100% effort – As required	– No reaction
12 – Full training	– Full training	– Gradually reintegrated	– No reaction

Figure 6.5 Return to running programme following hamstring injury.

No.	Exercise	Sets	Reps/ set	Load (kg)	Rest between sets	Speed of movt	Range of movt
1	VMO lunges Weight forward over front foot and hold lunge	3	12	Body weight	1 min	1-10-1-3	M
2	Single leg BOSU balance Unlock knee	5	1 x 30 s hold	–	Alternate legs	–	–
3	Step up onto box and then lower in front. Only FWB on standing leg and touch other toes down	3	12	Body weight	1 min	1-1-1-1	M
4	Glutes in standing at wall	10	1 x 10 s hold	–	Alternate legs	–	Iso
5	Knee drives	3	20	Body weight	1 min	1-0-1-0	F
6	BOSU forward hops	3	10 x 3 s hold	–	30 s	–	–
7	Walk through lunges	3	10	Body weight	1 min	–	F
8	Glute – hip extensions	3	15	–	1 min	1-0-1-0	F

Figure 6.6 Knee rehabilitation programme.

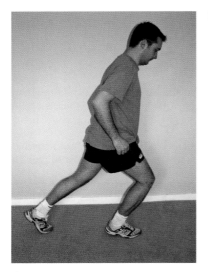

Figure 6.7 The VMO lunge.

No.	Exercise	Sets	Reps/ set	Load (kg)	Rest between sets	Speed of movt	Range of movt
1	VMO lunge pulses Weight forward over front foot and small knee flexion pulses	3	25	Body weight	1 min	1-0-1-0	M
2	BOSU forward hops	3	1 x 3 s hold	–	30 s	–	–
3	Glutes at wall – knee flex pulses Small knee flex pulses whilst maintaining glutes	3	20 pulses	Body weight	1 min	1-0-1-0	M
4	Step-up and overs	3	12	20 kg	1 min	2-1-2-1	F
5	Knee drives	3	30	Body weight	1 min	1-0-1-0	F
6	BOSU lateral hops	3	10 x 3 s hold	–	30 s	–	–
7	Jump lunges	3	20	Body weight	1 min	1-0-1-0	F
8	Glute – hip extensions	3	25	–	1 min	1-0-1-0	F

Figure 6.8 Late stage of rehabilitation process.

A similar programme can be used at the latter stages of the rehabilitation process with increases in repetitions to build endurance and making the proprioceptive exercises more difficult (Fig. 6.8).

Hamstring injuries

The hamstring muscles are the most commonly injured soft tissue and injury can cause athletes a significant time out of competitive play. They also have a high recurrence rate, with the biggest pre-disposing factor to a hamstring injury being a history of previous injury.

It has therefore been an area of great interest to ascertain the exact mechanism of injury occurring, how to rehabilitate the injury and also how to prevent the injury.

The injury tends to occur in one of two phases in the gait cycle:

1. The push-off phase, where the hamstring works concentrically to extend the hip to give a powerful push-off to sprint.
2. At the end of the swing phase, where the hamstring is working eccentrically to slow the leg down and specifically control the knee extension component. This is often compromised further where there is catching involved in

the sport, such as in rugby. It occurs when the athlete has to flex forward to catch the ball at the same time as slowing down which puts the hamstring on a stretch at the same time as working eccentrically.

Therefore, two key components of a hamstring rehabilitation programme are concentric hip extension strengthening exercises together with eccentric hamstring exercises which particularly concentrate on controlling knee extension.

The hamstring's other main function is to concentrically knee flex but this is not a movement that the hamstring has to work powerfully to do during running and therefore it is suggested that sports medics move away from purely strengthening the hamstring with resisted knee flexion exercises as it is not a functional movement for most athletes.

Consequently, there has been a lot written about the Nordic hamstring exercise. Here the athlete kneels with the feet fixed and slowly leans forward from the knees. Their hamstrings are required to work very hard eccentrically to control the movement. Some studies have shown that teams who have implemented a Nordic programme for their athletes in pre-season have significantly reduced their hamstring injury rates. This exercise can therefore be considered useful in preventing injuries, although one has to consider that it works in mid-knee flexion range, which is not in a functional position. It, therefore, should not become the 'be-all and end-all' to hamstring programmes and simply be part of an overall programme which addresses all the functional aspects required.

A list of progressive hamstring exercises with possible numbers of repetitions is listed below:

1. Hip extension drives
   - Attach T-band under arch/ball of foot, and other end to weight machine at head height
   - Start with hip flexed (band on that foot) to 90°, standing on other leg
   - Drive foot backwards to touch toes on foot behind stance leg
   - ×10 reps ×2 sets (Fig. 6.9).
2. Running motion – T-band kicks
   - Hook T-band under arch of foot
   - Tie opposite end of band to weights machine in front at head height
   - Circular running motion, focusing on push back
   - ×12 circles, ×3 sets
     - Increase speed with time (Fig. 6.10).
3. Glutes standing at wall
   - Stand side on to the wall, inside hip flexed to 90°, knee flexed to 90°
   - Push inside knee (bent knee) into wall
   - Turn standing leg out from the hip using glutes
   - Hold ×10 s, ×10 reps, ×2 sets (Fig. 6.11).
4. Forward gym ball drive
   - Gym ball is at chest height against wall
   - Straighten knee, drive ball up wall
   - ×10 reps, ×2 sets (Fig. 6.12).
5. Knee drives
   - Stand on one leg, other leg behind in hip extension
   - Drive free leg through in running style
   - Go up onto toes of standing leg
   - ×20 reps ×3 sets (Fig. 6.13).
6. Glute med sidelying (short lever)
   - Lie on one side, knees bent up, hand on back to keep still
   - Keep heels together, lift top knee turning out from hip
   - Lift heel off 2.5 cm, but maintain turn out of leg
   - Hold ×10 s ×10 reps ×3 sets (Fig. 6.14).

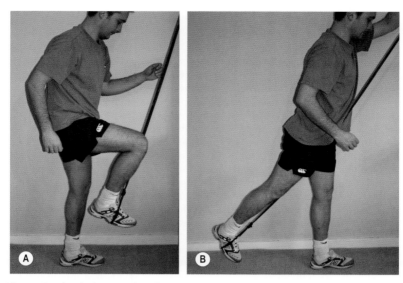

Figure 6.9 (A,B) Hip extension drives.

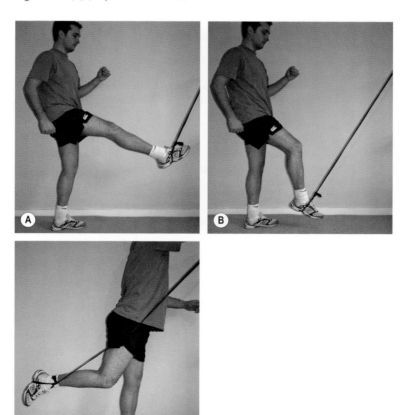

Figure 6.10 (A,B,C) Running motion T-band kicks.

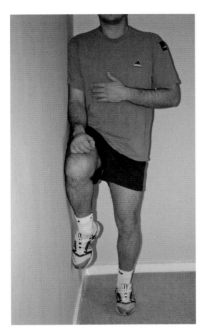

Figure 6.11 Glutes in stand at wall.

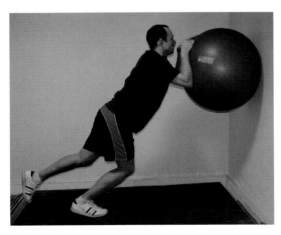

Figure 6.12 Forward gym ball drive.

7. Single-leg squats on Shuttle MVP
   - Lie on back on Shuttle MVP, one leg on plate
   - Push away quickly to straighten knee
   - Slow control on way back into knee bent
   - ×10 reps ×3 sets
     - Increase spring resistance (Fig. 6.15).
8. Bridging
   - Lie flat on your back on the floor, affected foot on the floor or a BOSU ball
   - Knee bent to start
   - Lift your buttocks off the floor and slowly lower

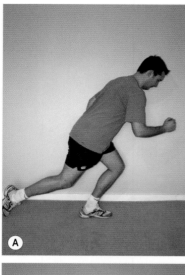
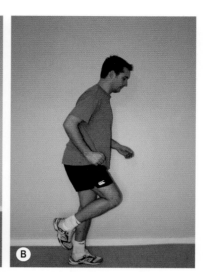
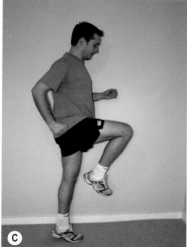

Figure 6.13 (A,B,C) Knee drives.

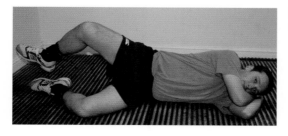

Figure 6.14 Gluteal clam.

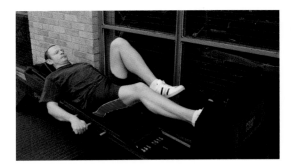

Figure 6.15 Single-leg squats on Shuttle MVP.

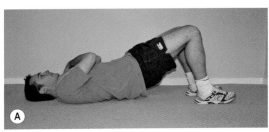

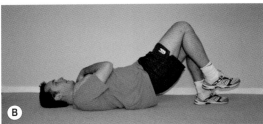

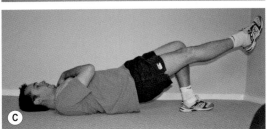

Figure 6.16 (A,B,C) Bridging.

- ×10 reps ×3 sets
  - Gradually straighten knees on sets of reps
  - Progress to holds ×5–10 s (Fig. 6.16).
9. Hip extension, standing on MVP
  - Standing, one foot on handle of MVP in slight hip extension and knee flexion. Just hold platform for balance
  - Push MVP back into hip extension
  - Slow return to start position
  - ×10 reps ×3 sets
    - Increase spring resistance as progression (Fig. 6.17).

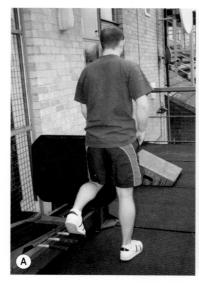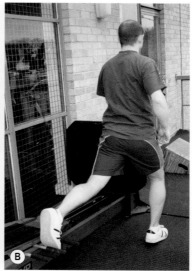

Figure 6.17 (A,B) Hip extension in standing on MVP.

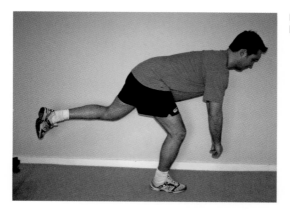

Figure 6.18 Forward lean.

10. Forward leans
    • Single-leg standing
    • Slight squat/knee bend, then flex forward from hips, keeping back straight, to touch floor with hands
    • ×10 slow reps ×3 sets
      ■ Progress to doing this holding medicine ball (Fig. 6.18).
11. Walk lunges
    • Walk through deep lunges with full drive up onto toes
    • Hold up-on-toes ×2 s, then back down into lunge
    • 6 widths of gym ×3 sets (Fig. 6.19).
12. Low passing with medicine ball
    • Standing, knees bent and full hip flex to lean forwards
    • Low passing both directions of medicine ball
    • 10 passes each direction
      ■ Progress to same exercise on BOSU ball (Fig. 6.20).

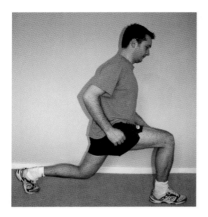

Figure 6.19 Walk lunges.

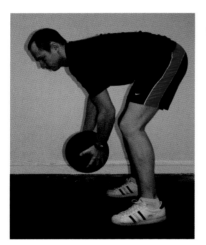

Figure 6.20 Low passing with medicine ball.

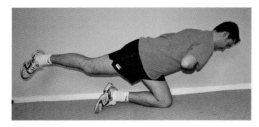

Figure 6.21 Kneeling forward leans.

13. Kneeling forward leans
- Kneel on plinth on 1 leg, other leg hanging off bed
- Bend knee to sit back on heel
- Then bend forwards from hips
- ×10 reps ×3 sets
  - Progress to holding medicine ball (Fig. 6.21).
14. T-band knee drives
- Tie band around ankle
- Attach other end of band to weights machine behind at low level

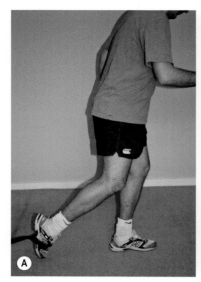 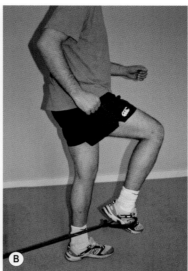

Figure 6.22 (A,B) T-band knee drives.

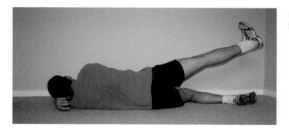

Figure 6.23 Glutes med side-lying (long lever).

- Drive leg forward with knee drive in running action
- Go up onto toes on standing leg, with opposite arm drive
- ×10 reps, ×3 sets (Fig. 6.22).

15. Glutes med side-lying (long lever)
- Knees straight, hips in slight extension, turning foot up to point upwards
- Ensure flat/neutral Lx spine is maintained throughout
- Abduct hip in laterally rotated and hip extended position
- Hold ×10 s, ×10 reps ×2 sets (Fig. 6.23).

16. Hip extension/glutes on gym ball
- Lie on your back on the floor, feet up onto gym ball
- Pull heels down into gym ball, lifting backside off floor
- Hold ×10 s, ×10 reps, ×2 sets
  - Progress to lifting alternate heels off gym ball (Fig. 6.24).

17. Hamstring curls in standing
- Tie T-band to foot/ankle and other end at floor level to something
- Bend knee up and slow return to knee straight
- ×12 reps, ×3 sets (Fig. 6.25).

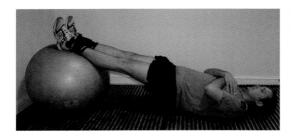

Figure 6.24 Hip extension.

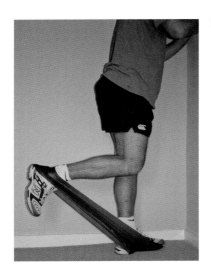

Figure 6.25 Hamstring curls in standing.

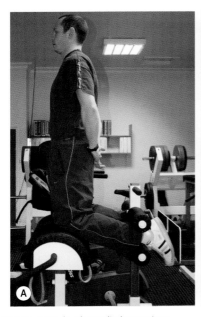

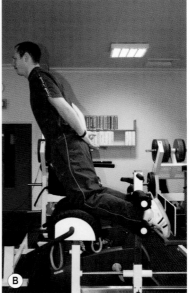

Figure 6.26 (A,B) Nordic hamstrings.

No.	Exercise	Sets	Reps/ set	Load (kg)	Rest between sets	Speed of movt	Range of movt
1	Theraband resisted eversion	3	12	Black Tband	1 min	2-1-2-1	F
2	Single leg BOSU balance	5	1 x 30 s hold	–	Alternate legs	–	–
3	Calf raises – straight knee	3	12	Body weight	1 min	1-1-2-1	F
4	BOSU forward hops	3	10 x 3 s hold	–	30 s	–	–
5	Calf raises – bent knee	3	12	Body weight	1 min	1-1-2-1	F
6	BOSU single leg squats	3	12	Body weight	1 min	1-0-1-0	M
7	Knee drives	3	20	Body weight	1 min	1-0-1-0	F
8	Glutes in standing at wall	10	1 x 10 s hold	–	Alternate legs	–	Iso

Figure 6.27 Ankle rehabilitation programme.

18. Jump lunges
    - From lunge, push up explosively to jump and alternate lunge
    - ×20 reps ×3 sets.
19. Nordic hamstrings – knees at 90°
    - Partner holds heels down
    - Player keeps arms crossed, core switched on, hips stay still
    - Straighten the knees by leaning forward using the hamstrings to control the movement. Drop to the floor when you cannot control with your hamstrings any more.
    - ×6 reps, ×3 sets (Fig. 6.26).

The Shuttle MVP is a cross between a leg press and a Pilates Reformer. It is spring loaded rather than using weights but provides a similar movement pattern to a leg press.

Ankle sprains

Ankle sprains and, in particular, lateral ligament sprains, are common injuries in a variety of sports that have a running or weight-bearing component.

Figure 6.27 is an example of a rehabilitation programme for an athlete who has suffered such an injury and is in the mid-stages of their rehabilitation.

Chapter | 7 |

Exercise and illness

© 2009 Elsevier Ltd, Inc, BV
DOI: 10.1016/B978-0-443-06813-3.00010-7

EXERCISE AND RESPIRATORY DISEASE

Dysfunction of the respiratory system plays an integral role in performance during exercise. It may well be that some of these symptoms are not attributable purely to respiratory pathology and there may be either an alternative or an overlap diagnosis with cardiac disease. Breathlessness is a common symptom during exercise, especially when the patient is sub-optimally fit or exercising intensely. However, if the patient complains of excessive shortness of breath or difficulty breathing, particularly at rest or at low intensity exercise, then there may be a pathological condition going on. It may also be that the patient complains of difficulty in breathing when performing some exercise that they do not normally have any trouble with and this may become more apparent in different environmental conditions.

The most common cause of breathlessness is exercise-induced asthma. However, there may be other causes which need to be excluded and these include respiratory infections, spontaneous pneumothorax or foreign body aspiration as well as chronic obstructive airways disease. Non-respiratory causes such as cardiac ischaemia or valve disease, pulmonary embolus and anaemia as well as obesity and psychological causes need to be excluded.

A diagnosis is made by taking a full history and examination and performing investigations including respiratory function tests (see below), chest X-ray, ECG and blood tests to exclude the causes mentioned above.

Difficulty in breathing is often associated with a wheeze which, by definition, is described as an expiratory noise as opposed to an inspiratory stridor, which may reflect upper airway obstruction. Wheeze is often a symptom of bronchospasm but be aware that the patient may not need to have wheeze nor difficulty in breathing to be diagnosed as asthmatic. Some asthmatics just have a cough that may be present at night time or triggered off by exercise. The nature of the cough, being productive or non-productive or being during the day or night, may have a reflection on the diagnosis and possible causes include post-nasal drip and sinusitis, reflux oesophagitis and aspiration or bronchogenic carcinoma and including the differential diagnoses mentioned above.

Some patients complain of chest pain or tightness and obviously cardiac ischaemia needs to be excluded in these patients but this may also be the exhibiting symptom of exercise-induced asthma or bronchospasm as well as symptoms that may affect the chest wall such as rib injuries, costovertebral and costosternal joint injuries, referred pain from the thoracic spine and early onset herpes zoster.

Intercostal muscle injuries as well as pleuritic chest infections can also present this way.

Investigation, as listed above, is needed to make a differential.

Asthma

Asthma is a chronic inflammatory disease of the airways as a result of hyper-reactivity resulting in various symptoms to include coughing, wheezing, chest tightness and shortness of breath. The cough may be dry, irritating and persistent, often worse in the morning or late at night or after exercise and this is due to a mixture of variable airway obstruction, variable reversible airway obstruction and associated inflammation within the bronchii. Allergic triggers include house-dust mite, pollens, fungi and animal allergens but other triggers also include upper respiratory tract infections, exercise and emotional triggers including stress and laughter, as well as changes in temperature and humidity. As mentioned above, the absence of a wheeze does not exclude the diagnosis of asthma.

Exercise-induced asthma (EIA) occurs when there is bronchospasm rather than mucus overproduction and inflammation as a result of exercise. Most commonly, this occurs at the completion of exercise rather than during it and it is the exercise that triggers the bronchospasm rather than any other allergic trigger. It is estimated that 10% of the general population have symptoms associated with exercise-induced asthma and it is possible for an asthmatic to have exercise-induced asthma as well as his background asthma.[1-3]

The pathogenesis of exercise-induced asthma is controversial and may be a result of change in humidity or temperature of inhaled air. During exercise, most athlete's mouth-breathe, thus bypassing the normal humidification processes that occurs in the nose. This results in relative dehydration of the inhaled air which seems to trigger off bronchospasm.

Asthma and exercise-induced asthma are diagnosed through respiratory function tests. The simplest test of this is measuring FEV1; the amount of forced expiratory volume within 1 s, as measured by a spirometer. By definition, asthma and exercise-induced asthma are reversible airways obstruction and so with both of these, one would expect to see a reduction in the FEV1 of greater than 12%, with exercise only to be reversible with bronchodilators such as salbutamol. The degree of drop in FEV1 or peak expiratory flow rate, as measured on a peak flow-meter, reflects the severity of the asthma. Other forms of diagnostic criteria include a eucapnic voluntary hyperpnoea test, which involves hyperventilation with dry air containing 0.9% carbon dioxide at varying levels of maximum voluntary ventilation and demonstrating a drop of FEV1 by more than 10%, which is then reversible again on the use of a bronchodilator.

Various studies have shown that anything between 9% and 15% of athletes are shown to have an undiagnosed exercise-induced asthma.

Treatment of asthma includes management of the inflammatory component, usually by a corticosteroid inhaler, and reversing the bronchospasm with bronchodilator inhalers. Both these medications need to be notified through a therapeutic usage exemption (TUE) form or declaration of use notification for the use of drug testing.

Management of exercise-induced asthma, however, involves the avoidance of exercising in a dry or cold environment, although this is not always possible. The use of masks or nose-breathing regimes have proved less effective. It is important, perhaps, that there is gradual warming up towards 80–90% of maximum intensity, so as to decrease the change in environmental factors affecting the airways; however, the mainstay of the treatment is the use of bronchodilators within the first 15 min of activity to try and counter the bronchospasm. If this is ineffective, then the use of alternative treatments, including inhaled corticosteroids, leuko-triene receptor antagonists and long-acting beta-agonists, have been used.

EXERCISE AND CARDIOVASCULAR DISEASE

There are always concerns when advising patients with cardiovascular disease as to how they should best exercise, and, before giving advice, it is important to understand what changes occur in the cardiovascular system with exercise.

With exercise, the heart responds by increasing its rate and contractility and with long-term exercise, resistance training can lead to pressure overload, whereas endurance training can lead to volume overload.

With pressure overload there is an increase in septal and free wall ventricular thickness, whereas in volume overload, such as in distance running athletes, there is left ventricular end diastolic diameter increase with a proportionate increase in the ventricular wall thickness.

Patients who combine weight training with endurance have a mixture of these two changes. As a result, athletes may present with a heart that is either normal size but has thickened walls or has a larger sized ventricle with a proportional increase in wall thickness or a combination of the two. It is obviously important to distinguish these changes from both pathological changes and, likewise, it is the changes that are not uncommon on examining an athlete. It is not unusual to find a slow resting pulse and an increased left ventricular size with an apex beat displaced laterally in a normal athlete. Systolic murmurs are not uncommon but it would be abnormal to find a raised blood pressure, a raised JVP or peripheral oedema. Likewise, ECG changes are not uncommon in an athlete, with sinus bradycardia and left ventricular hypertrophy being regarded as normal in 80% of athletes, and ST segment elevation is not uncommon. However, other rhythm abnormalities such as atrial fibrillation or heart block cannot necessarily be attributable to the patient being an athlete.

Bearing this in mind, what symptoms would be regarded as abnormal in an athlete when they may have cardiovascular disease?

Symptoms of palpitations, chest pain or syncopal attacks or dizzy attacks would be regarded as abnormal. Likewise, a family history or a history of murmurs needs to be investigated.

Palpitations

It is important when a patient presents with palpitations to be absolutely sure that this is what they are describing and not some fasciculation in their chest wall muscles or a feeling of anxiety. Other cardiac symptoms, such as chest pain, dizziness and syncope, need to be excluded and then if you are sure that they have palpitations you need to determine their onset, their triggers, their duration and whether they are regular or irregular in nature.

A history of medication, recreational drug abuse, eating disorders or other cardiac events needs to be excluded as well as other triggers, such as thyroid disease, hypoglycemia, caffeinated drinks and ephedrine. Remember that some athletes take pseudoephedrine or caffeine as a pick-me-up before competing and these can stimulate the heart.

Examination must exclude thyroid disease, cardiac murmur or an arrhythmia. Chest X-ray and ECG are helpful but it may be that the athlete needs to precipitate an attack with an exercise regime using an exercise test on a treadmill or wearing a halter monitoring system. If an abnormal exercise test results, then an echocardiogram needs to be performed to exclude an underlying structural abnormality.

It is beyond the boundaries of this book to go into the treatment of cardiac arrhythmias but it is important to be aware that no cardiac structural abnormality should be omitted. It is also worthwhile being aware that the treatment for some of the cardiac arrhythmias includes beta blockers which are on WADA's list of banned substances in certain sports, as by reducing the cardiac rate they may provide an advantage in precision sports such as shooting.

Syncope or dizzy attacks

Syncope is the loss of postural tone with an inability to stand upright and loss of consciousness brought about by reduction in cerebral blood flow due to reduced cardiac output. It is often associated with nausea and vomiting and the patient often looks pale or grey with cold sweat. The symptoms are similar when the patient is anaemic or hypoglycemic or when there is cerebral ischaemia such as from TIAs. However, it can occur with cardiac output abnormalities resulting in postural hypotension. It is important to determine whether this occurs during or after sport as syncope or fainting immediately after an event could be due to pooling of blood in the lower limbs because of absence of muscle contractility and the muscle pump pushing the blood back into the heart, reducing cardiac output and this has been labelled as exercise-associated collapse.[4]

Treatment is with head down and leg elevation and recovery is quick; however, if the athlete has syncopal attacks during sporting activities this can indicate a medical problem and should be taken seriously. A full history including family history of cardiac events or sudden death at a young age and a history excluding diabetes, valvular disease and hypertension needs to be excluded as well as other symptoms of cardiac disease as mentioned above. A full cardiac examination and investigations including chest X-ray, ECG, exercise stress testing echocardiogram need to be performed.

Syncope can easily be dismissed as a dizzy attack or a funny feeling and sometimes this can be confused with vertigo or hypoglycaemia. It is important for the doctor to be aware that this can be the one and only symptom that the athlete can complain of that can give you a pointer towards some underlying cardiac abnormality and it is vital to be alert to this symptom and to investigate it appropriately.

Sudden cardiac death

Sudden cardiac death related to exercise is fortunately not common but often has a high profile, as it is so tragic in occurring in otherwise fit and healthy athletes.[5-7]

Although exercising substantially reduces the risk of cardiac death, in those who are susceptible, intense exercise may increase their particular risk. Sudden death is divided into two age groups: those under the age of 35 who show evidence of a structural, congenital cardiovascular lesion and those over 35 who die of coronary artery disease. Sudden death in the young is a tragic event and in several countries around the world there are screening programmes to identify those at risk. Within the UK, CRY (Cardiac Risk in the Young) is a society that provides advice, screening and counselling for those who are at risk from this condition.

Unfortunately, there are many athletes whose first symptom of cardiac disease is their sudden death and every week eight apparently fit and healthy young people die in the UK from undiagnosed heart conditions. The most common cause of sudden death in athletes is hypertrophic cardiomyopathy which accounts for 36% of deaths in one study. This condition is characterised by hypertrophy of the ventricular wall and is associated with either an obstruction or nonobstruction to the left ventricular out-flow. It is more common in males and most sufferers have no symptoms prior to the tragic event. However, of those that did have symptoms, the most common was exertional dyspnoea which should not be confused with asthma, chest pain, or palpitations as well as pre-syncope or pseudo-syncopal attacks. Patients with hypertrophic cardiomyopathy have a jerky, carotid pulse with a double or triple apex beat associated with a cardiac murmur. There is often a fourth heart sound but otherwise examination may be normal. ECG shows evidence of left ventricular hypertrophy, ST segment changes and prominent Q waves, although, as said previously, these signs may be found in a normal athlete. However, a normal ECG makes a diagnosis of hypertrophic cardiomyopathy unlikely.

Diagnosis is clinched through an echocardiogram showing a hypertrophied non-dilated left ventricle with an absolute thickness of the left ventricle wall greater than 15 mm. It is this measurement that determines the difference between a hypertrophic cardiomyopathy and an athlete's heart and it is important that the echocardiogram is performed by an experienced ultrasonographer. CRY offer screening programmes to adolescents and this is a service that is being increasingly used whereby the athletes are given a questionnaire exploring symptoms and family histories and then arranged to have an examination and an ECG. Those that have any positive answers on questionnaires, examination or have some abnormalities on ECG are offered an echocardiogram. In Italy, all children have to have this screening test to be allowed to proceed to a sport in their team; however, it is a highly expensive screening programme with very little pick-up unless you are the athlete that is found to have this condition.

As a sports physician, it is important to be aware of the warning symptoms so that these patients can be identified and investigated appropriately.

Cardiac murmurs

Heart murmurs are not uncommon in the athletic heart and it is the role of the sports physician to determine whether these are innocent or significant. An innocent flow murmur is usually short and systolic, unlike the harsh murmur of aortic stenosis radiating to the neck. All diastolic murmurs require further investigation with an ECG and echocardiogram.

Chest pain

It is not uncommon for athletes to present with chest pain and it is important for the sports physician to think beyond the musculoskeletal causes of this.

Causes such as rib pathology, costovertebral and costosternal joint pains, intercostal muscle injuries, referred pain from the thoracic spine, respiratory causes and dermatological causes such as herpes zoster need to be excluded. However, cardiac causes also need to be excluded, such as cardiac ischaemia and pericarditis, as well as pulmonary emboli.

Marfan's syndrome

It is important to also mention Marfan's syndrome which is an autosomal dominant condition found in 0.02% of the population.[8]

Family history is often negative, although it is dominant as it is usually caused by new mutations. These patients present with multi-system disease mainly affecting the eyes, cardiac system and musculoskeletal system. Their main worry is one of aortic root aneurysm rupture causing sudden death; however, they also suffer from tall stature, wide arm span, chest deformities, hypermobility, cardiac murmur including mitral valve prolapse and regurgitation and myopia.

Ironically, it is some of these features that make them particularly well adapted for sport, including basketball and volleyball.

Examination may show a high arched palate, wide arm span and hyperflexible joints and investigations in a patient suspected of having Marfan's syndrome should include a chest X-ray, which may show aortic dilatation, and more importantly echocardiogram. It is not uncommon to see patients with this condition in a sports injury clinic and the physician needs to be aware of this condition.

Screening for sudden death

Of the list of conditions that may cause sudden death or cardiac disease, which criteria are useful in deciding which patients to investigate?

The following can be used as a guideline:

1. Sudden death under the age of 35 in a first degree relative
2. Exercise-induced or unexplained syncopal symptoms, dyspnoea, palpitations or chest pain
3. First degree relative with hypertrophic cardiomyopathy or Marfan's syndrome
4. Examination findings that include a diastolic murmur or a new cardiac systolic murmur or new onset arrhythmia.

Take home points

- Exercise-induced asthma is not uncommon in otherwise fit elite athletes.
- Cough may be the only symptom of asthma.
- Important cardiac symptoms may be very subtle in athletes, so spend time getting a clear and accurate history.

EXERCISE AND GASTROINTESTINAL ILLNESS

It is well known that exercise can bring about some physiological changes in the gastrointestinal (GI) tract, such as alteration in gastric emptying and intestinal mobility, as well as variation in blood flow to the GI tract. As a result there can be an association with variation in appetite, an increasing incidence of heartburn, reflux oesophagitis and chest pain, associated with belching, vomiting and nausea. There can be increased intestinal hurry with diarrhoea, abdominal cramping and, at times, rectal bleeding.

Dyspepsia

Under this umbrella, the symptoms of nausea, vomiting, reflux, heartburn, belching and trapped wind can be included. It is well known that patients, who have these symptoms without exercise, tend to get an exacerbation with exercise. It is important to be absolutely sure that these symptoms are, first confined to the GI tract and are not a symptom of cardiovascular or respiratory cause of chest pain, such as ischaemia, arrhythmia or respiratory dysfunction, in addition to excluding any musculoskeletal cause in the chest, such as costosternal joint dysfunction or referred pain from the thoracic spine. Be aware that the gastric emptying rate may be increased with exercise, although other factors, such as meal volume and content, as well as a level of anxiety within the athlete can play a role. It is therefore important to reduce the distention of the stomach during exercise and, if possible, one should avoid solid food for 3 h before intense exercise and the pre-match meal should be high in carbohydrate and low in protein and fat. Antacids, H2 receptor antagonists and even PPIs play a role in reducing the acidity within the stomach. Likewise, domperidone 1 h before meals can be effective. Be aware that some athletes take antiinflammatories, either long-term or before exercise or competition and this may have a negative effect on dyspepsia.[9]

GI bleeding, whether it is from the upper GI tract or lower GI tract, must be taken seriously, and pathological conditions excluded before it is presumed it is due to exercise. Alterations in blood flow affecting ischaemic colitis as well as the effect of antiinflammatories can all result in rectal bleeding, which should be investigated. Also, remember that chronic low level asymptomatic GI bleeding can result in anaemia and low ferritin levels, which can be a cause of decreased performance and fatigue. Serum ferritin levels of less than 30 ng/mL in women and 50 ng/mL in men indicate reduced iron stores.

Diarrhoea

As mentioned above, this is not an uncommon symptom of exercise.[10] It may be related to the intensity of exercise rather than the exercise itself. With any episode of diarrhoea other causes need to be excluded, such as infected diarrhoea, be it viral or bacterial. In most cases this can be treated expectantly with prevention of dehydration, possible isolation if the patient is a team player involved in close contact with other team members, good hygiene and the avoidance of solid food while maintaining carbohydrate intake and monitoring progress until the diarrhoea settles down. Most cases can be treated without medication; however, in an urgent case prior to competition, it has been known for either ciprofloxacin 1 g or norfloxacin 800 mg in a stat dose to be prescribed, together with loperamide 4 mg titrated against the frequency of diarrhoea to provide rapid symptom relief and allow an athlete to perform. Generally speaking, however, loperamide should not be a routine form of treatment. Other causes of diarrhoea need to be excluded, such as excessive fibre intake, other forms of medication such as supplements, caffeine or sweeteners. Likewise, it is important to exclude other lower GI pathological conditions, such as, colitis, colonic polyps and irritable bowel syndrome. Persistent diarrhoea needs to be investigated with stool microscopy and blood test to exclude anaemia, inflammatory bowel disease and coeliac disease, as well as colonoscopy and possibly biopsy.

Irritable bowel disease

This condition is very common in the non-exercise population, and therefore, it is not surprising to find it in those who exercise. It has a close association with anxiety and emotional levels, and therefore sometimes can present only at competition. The symptoms can vary from distention, abdominal pain, flatulence and belching, constipation and diarrhoea, sometimes alternating, but rectal bleeding should not be put down to irritable bowel syndrome (IBS) unless otherwise investigated. This can be a difficult condition to treat as it may only present a few hours before competition. However, if an athlete is susceptible to this condition it would be worthwhile looking at their diet and altering the roughage content, or experimenting with the use of either regular or pre-exercise antispasmodics, such as, Colofac, or peppermint tablets.

Abdominal pain

As has been mentioned above, exercise can affect the GI tract in many ways and abdominal pain is not uncommon. It is important, however, to make sure abdominal pain is definitely coming from the GI tract and not from any musculoskeletal cause, such as, thoracolumbar referred pain, psoas pathology or indeed any urinary or gynaecological cause. Within the exercise population a stitch is a common cause of abdominal pain, the cause of which is not fully known; spasm of the diaphragm or trapping of distended gas within the hepatic or splenic flexure have been postulated, as well as the theory that exercising too close to a meal may cause this pain. However, it is not exactly known what causes this.

EXERCISE AND ENT CONDITIONS

Otalgia

Earache is not uncommon in the sporting population and a good knowledge of possible good differential diagnoses is important. Most commonly it is due to an otitis media associated with an upper respiratory tract infection, of which the majority settle down with supportive treatment and analgesia. Rarely are antibiotics required; however, it is recognised in the athletic population that there is often urgency, and a pressure to treat these patients more aggressively and therefore, at times, antibiotics may be indicated. Other causes of otalgia include pressure changes within the middle ear, associated with eustachian tube dysfunction, which can be precipitated by foreign travel and arrow trauma. Pain referred from the temporomandibular joint (TMJ) can present as earache; however, this is easy to diagnose as the TMJ is often tender and there is discomfort on mastication or moving the mandible. A palpable click is sometimes felt on opening and closing the mouth. Referred pain from the cervical spine or neck musculature, including the sternomastoid and trapezius can cause earache; however, do not forget that herpes zoster (Ramsay Hunt syndrome) can present as severe earache and often there are no external dermatological signs apart from one or two blisters that may only be present in the external auditory meatus.

The most common cause of earache in swimmers is otitis externa, otherwise known as swimmer's ear or tropical ear. It is an infection of the external auditory canal. Whether this is a primary infection, either with *Staphylococcus aureus* or *Pseudomonas,* or added infection on top of an underlying eczema is not really clear; however, the persistent wetting of the external auditory meatus seen either in swimmers or in patients in hot climates sets up an itch cycle clearly seen. The itching then causes further breaking up of the soggy mucosa within the external auditory meatus, which then allows infection. The patient can complain of severe pain around the ear associated with an itch and discharge. Movement of the ear is painful, as with eating, pulling on the tragus or pinna. The treatment includes suction toilet to remove any debris within the ear, keeping the ear dry, often with the use of a hairdryer and the application of antibiotic and cortisone-related eardrops. Analgesia is important as these conditions can be very painful, and occasionally, assessment by an ENT specialist is valuable.

Common cold

Sports physicians are often asked for advice on best management of the common cold or upper respiratory tract infection in athletic competitors. It is important not to make these patients dependent on antibiotic medication for what is generally a viral illness and self-limiting. Obviously, it is important to differentiate this from tonsillitis or infectious mononucleosis; however, generally speaking, these can be treated with symptomatic control involving rest, fluids, decongestants and gargles.

Infectious mononucleosis

Throat infections with the Epstein–Barr virus causing glandular fever are very common within the young athletic population. Adolescents typically develop a sore throat, malaise, headache and, less commonly, myalgia, nausea and flu-like illnesses. Examination will show a fever with pharyngitis and tonsillitis with swollen cervical and sometimes axillary lymph nodes. Typically, there is palatal petechiae, just anterior to the uvula. Splenomegaly occurs in 50% of cases and peaks in the second or third week of illness. A similar illness can be seen with cytomegalovirus and toxoplasmosis infections. The infection is infectious and although it is thought to be due to close contact in kissing, it can spread throughout a squad of players quickly. This condition therefore, needs to be confirmed serologically and the patient isolated. Treatment involves symptomatic treatment to reduce fever and sore throat and the avoidance of ampicillin or Amoxil-related drugs, as these can cause a macular rash.

Complications with infectious mononucleosis are as for any systemic illness and include avoidance of sport until all acute symptoms have resolved. The worry with infectious mononucleosis is the risk of splenic rupture due to the vulnerability of a hypertrophied swollen spleen. The risk of splenic rupture is maximum within the first 21 days of illness; the majority of which may be before the patient actually has symptoms. It is therefore important to restrict contact sport for the first 3 weeks of the known symptoms. Return to contact sport should be allowed once the patient is systemically well, the liver and spleen are no longer tender or palpably enlarged and the patient has had more than 3 weeks' duration of the illness. Delayed splenic rupture is recognised and a decision needs to be made on a case-by-case basis. Ultrasound scanning of the spleen can be useful although normal sizes of a spleen vary from patient to patient and it is unlikely that a preillness splenic ultrasound has been performed.

Nasal discharge and sinus pain

Sinusitis is defined as the occurrence of facial pain, be it in the maxillary, ethmoid or frontal sinuses, associated with fever, nasal discharge or post-nasal drip, and tenderness over the sinuses, which worsens on putting your head between your knees. The sinuses can become tender when they are congested, associated with an upper respiratory viral illness; however, true sinusitis is very different and can be very disabling. A history of broken nose can precipitate sinusitis, as can a history of perennial rhinitis or hay fever. Examination will show tenderness over the sinuses with a hyperaemic nasal passage and often post-nasal drip. Treatment includes symptomatic treatment involving paracetamol and steam inhalations but true sinusitis needs to be treated with antibiotics, and a good history needs to be taken to exclude an underlying chronic rhinitis that would benefit from inhaled nasal steroids.

Take home points

- Treat diarrhoea correctly – do not be tempted to treat with antibiotics and anti-diarrhoeal agents on a whim.
- Be familiar with the symptoms, signs and management of infectious mononucleosis.

EXERCISE AND DIABETES

This section on exercise and diabetes is not designed to be an extensive chapter on diabetes and the complications of this disease. Instead, this is meant to give an outline of the basics of diabetes and some advice on how a diabetic should adjust their medication in response to exercise and also what role exercise may play in causing complications in a diabetic.[11]

Type 1 diabetes is an inherited autoimmune disease where there is a lack of endogenous insulin production as a result of antibody production against the insulin-producing cells in the pancreas. Treatment is through insulin administration to prevent hyperglycaemia, ketoacidosis and death. The aim of treatment is to maintain a blood sugar level below 11 and an HbA1C below 7.0, with a view to, not only controlling the condition, but preventing the complications that ensue. These include effects on the cardiovascular system, such as hypertension and postural hypotension, reduction in peripheral blood flow and coronary artery disease. In addition, retinopathy, cataracts and glaucoma, as well as peripheral neuropathy and renal damage can occur, if there is suboptimal control.

Type 2 diabetes is more linked to lifestyle and genetic factors and results in insulin resistance and lack of sensitivity to insulin production, resulting in hyperglycaemia. This is a much more common cause of diabetes and is strongly linked to lack of exercise and obesity.[12]

For both a diabetic and a patient suffering from cardiovascular disease the aim is to be involved in at least 30 min of moderate exercise activity (either in the form of cycling or brisk walking) 5–6 days a week. Ideally, we are looking at increasing the heart rate to 60% of the maximum heart rate (maximum being 220 minus the patient's age), although bear in mind that those patients with complications, as a result of their diabetes, may have an autonomic neuropathy that may affect their heart rate. Exercise in an insulin-dependent diabetic has the effect of lowering the insulin requirements. In fact, the action of insulin and exercise is cumulative and a reduction in as much as 25–30% of insulin requirements has been seen with exercise. It is therefore important that those with diabetes monitor their blood sugar levels, both before and after every exercise session, and if the exercise session is unexpectedly altered by either prolonging it or shortening it, then this can have an unexpected effect on the blood sugar level. Likewise, changes in environmental issues and workload involved in training sessions can equally have a dramatic effect. Ideally a pre-exercise blood level of glucose should be between 6.5 and 10.0, but those with a blood sugar level less than 5.5 should supplement their sugar level with a pre-exercise carbohydrate snack until it is above 6.5. It is not a good idea for the patient to exercise with a blood sugar level above 16.5 until they have reduced their glucose level with extra insulin. Type 2 diabetics, on no oral medication, do not need to make any special adjustments with regard to exercise; however, those taking oral hypoglycaemics may need to reduce their dose by a quarter to a half on the days of prolonged exercise or even avoid taking the medication while still monitoring the sugar levels. It is obvious, therefore, that each diabetic should be familiar with the effect of exercise on their own blood sugar levels, and anticipate what effect this will have in advance.

The main risks of exercise in a diabetic athlete are those of hypoglycaemia, with a blood sugar less than 3.6, either due to excess exercise or too much insulin. The typical symptoms of sweating, headache, nervousness, confusion and eventual collapse need to be identified early on and avoided, with oral carbohydrate, in the form of glucose tablets or glucose drinks. Glucose gels in the form of Hypostop are useful for those who are unconscious and cannot swallow; however, glucagon or intravenous 50% glucose solution is the treatment of choice.

Diabetics are also at risk of other musculoskeletal ailments and these include carpal tunnel syndrome, Dupuytren's contracture, and adhesive capsulitis of the shoulder.

EXERCISE AND EPILEPSY

Epilepsy is defined as a neurological brain disorder resulting in recurrent seizures. It is important to recognise that recurrent means more than two seizures, as single seizures, including those as a result of a head injury, febrile convulsions and trauma-related convulsions do not constitute epilepsy. It is beyond the scope of this text to go into great detail about epilepsy but enough to say that seizures in an individual can be the result of an underlying epilepsy or some other condition. Epilepsy itself can be defined into seizures that are either generalised or focal and are complex or partial. Generalised epileptic seizures involve the whole body with chronic body movements whereas focal epilepsy originates from one localised area within the brain causing a localised physical convulsion. Complex or partial seizures denote whether consciousness is lost or not.

Seizures that are not due to epilepsy consist of syncopal convulsions that may occur as a result of hypotensive attacks due to cardiovascular or metabolic causes such as hypoglycemia and traumatic events, mainly in the form of head injuries most commonly seen as a concussive convulsion which are a benign phenomena and do not require further investigation. It is important in these latter patients to be absolutely sure that the convulsion is the confirmed diagnosis rather than there being a head injury with some underlying brain injury and a thorough neurological examination with or without imaging may be appropriate. Any doubt about the diagnosis can be confirmed on an EEG with or without neuro-imaging in the form of an MRI.[13]

Exercise in epileptics should be encouraged, although the seizure frequency may be affected by this, both in a positive and a negative way. However, it is important to realise that some forms of activity should be performed with caution in people who have epilepsy. Epileptics who have frequent and unpredictable seizures should be advised not to perform in scuba diving, rock climbing, parachuting or horseback riding. Likewise, downhill ski racing and sports that involve operating machinery such as racing car driving would have certain restrictions. In activities that involve being in isolation, such as orienteering or possibly swimming, these athletes should be warned that they should be performing with a buddy just in case they have a seizure that needs attention. It should also be noted that there are certain legal requirements to be fulfilled in patients with epilepsy when driving a car (refer to the DVLA guidelines).

Generally speaking, however, there are very few restrictions on epilepsy; however, team physicians, coaches and possibly team members should be informed of this player's situation with the patient's consent so that there is no fear about dealing with a potential problem and so that the general public are reassured that a healthy lifestyle can coexist with this condition.

EXERCISE AND JOINT PAINS

It is important for the sports physician to realise that there is significant overlap between the field of rheumatology and inflammatory disease and sports medicine.[14]

There are many conditions that can present initially in both fields of speciality, either as an Achilles tendinopathy to a sports physician's clinic that can be a tendinopathy manifestation of a systemic spondyloarthropathy, and conversely, a de Quervain's tenosynovitis that may be an overuse injury in a squash player. It is within the remit of the sports physician to always be on the lookout for 'sports injuries' that are a manifestation of a more systemic or inflammatory condition. Injuries that do not fit the usual cause or pattern, with significant night pain or stiffness, or are associated with a past or present history of other manifestations, need to be investigated. Likewise, no convincing history of injury or trauma or overuse needs to be dealt with, with an open mind.

There are many inflammatory causes of single or multiple joint pains as well as pains affecting the lumbar spine. However, it is probably sensible to divide them into three main categories:

1. Monoarthropathy (single swollen joint pain)
2. Polyarthropathy (multiple swollen joint pain)
3. Low back pain and stiffness with or without other joint pain.

Monoarthropathy

Single joint pain is not uncommon in both fields of sports medicine and inflammatory joint disease and the physician should have a high index of suspicion especially when there is no obvious trauma or overuse. A warm, red, swollen, painful joint with some morning stiffness and night pain should raise suspicions of either an inflammatory, infected or neoplastic condition.

The physician should therefore explore other causes and stigmata of inflammatory disease such as:

1. Skin conditions including psoriatic arthritis associated with nail dystrophy, insertional tendon enthesopathy, low back pain and the characteristic rash most classical in the periumbilical and sacral area as well as over the knees and elbows
2. A history of bowel disorder including ulcerative colitis and Crohn's disease suggesting enteropathic arthropathy
3. Rheumatological conditions such as rheumatoid arthritis where there is symmetrical polyarthropathy of the small joints of the hands, wrist and feet but in 15% present as single monoarthropathies
4. Reiter's disease including symptoms of urethral discharge and iritis
5. Gout or pseudo-gout, the former as a result of dietary indiscretions, renal disease or diuretic drug use and pseudo-gout as a result of calcium pyrophosphate deposits within the joint that are seen in association with hyperthyroidism and hyperparathyroidism
6. Septic arthritis as seen in those with impaired immunity and/or diabetes.

A significant proportion of these patients have a positive family history which needs to be explored. Examination needs to be generalised to identify all the above stigmata and to give a pointer as to whether this is a particular inflammatory disorder.

Investigations help to confirm or refute an inflammatory, infective or neoplastic condition and most commonly include erythrocytes sedimentation rate (ESR) and C-reactive protein which are also helpful in the blood test quest, as are urethral swabs and stool swabs if enteropathic or Reiter's arthritis are suspected. The screening of other rheumatological blood tests such as rheumatoid factor, antinuclear antibodies and HLAB27 is contentious. Approximately 80% of patients with rheumatoid arthritis are rheumatoid factor positive but there is a 15% false positive finding when performing blanket screening. Likewise, antinuclear antibodies are almost 100% in patients with SLE but they are also found in patients with scleroderma, rheumatoid arthritis, other diseases of the thyroid, liver and lung as well as 15% of healthy people. HLAB27 is a normal gene found in 8% of healthy, normal individuals but is also associated with ankylosing spondylitis, psoriatic arthritis and enteropathic arthritis. It is therefore recommended that these three tests may give a significant false positive finding and should not be used routinely in blood tests.

Plain X-rays are sometimes useful to identify bone erosions and cysts, calcified tendons and to exclude tumours.

Treatment is with antiinflammatory modalities, both pharmacological and non-pharmacological; however, advice from a rheumatological specialist may be indicated if this condition does not settle quickly.

Polyarthropathy

The conditions that can cause an inflammatory monoarthropathy can also affect more than one joint at one time and most commonly these include rheumatoid arthritis which affects symmetrical joints, small joints of the hands, wrist and feet, mainly the PIP joints, MCP joints and MTP joints. Reactive polyarthropathy as found in genito-urinary and GI infections can occur asymmetrically in larger joints, mainly the knees and elbows, associated with enthesopathies of tendons. This occurs more rapidly in onset (in a matter of days) as opposed to over a period of weeks and months with rheumatoid arthritis. Psoriatic arthritis, inflammatory osteoarthrosis and systemic lupus erythematosus can all present with multiple joint inflammation.

Again, examination needs to be thorough and beyond a musculoskeletal basis and joint basis to include skin, eyes, tendons and even abdominal examination.

The investigations, not surprisingly, include ESR and C-reactive protein and further investigation and referral may be appropriate.

Low back pain and stiffness associated with joint arthropathy

Low back pain is a common reason for referral in sports injury clinics, and not infrequently, they present with an inflammatory spondyloarthropathy. This includes inflammatory arthritis of the spine and sacroiliac joints as a result of the inflammatory conditions that have been mentioned above. These patients are more likely to be HLAB27 positive although a negative result does not eliminate the diagnosis. It is more common in young, fit males aged below 30. Classically they present with low back pain which is worse at night with marked early morning stiffness of more than 2 h duration which is eased by antiinflammatories. This is not a mechanical low back pain.

Examination

The sports physician should be alert to a more generalised examination, especially when a patient describes low back pain with early morning stiffness. A general examination looking at peripheral as well as large joints, and looking specifically for the skin discoloration of lupus or psoriasis and evidence of calcific tendinopathy or iritis, is important not to miss. The physician should look for sacroiliac joint tenderness and pain on springing with restriction in lumbosacral lateral flexion followed by extension. In these cases, performing an HLAB27 may be appropriate.

X-rays may show evidence of sacroiliitis confirming ankylosing spondylitis as well as the bone spurs and bone bridging that is seen in a thoracolumbar ankylosing spondylitis. Early identification and management of these patients is important.

Other joint pains

Although not specific to inflammatory disease within this category there are patients who complain of multiple joint pains and pains all over, not just confined to the joints but other musculoskeletal tissues as well as other parts of the body. It can be challenging to manage these patients; however, as a summary the following causes need to be excluded:

- Viral illness including reactions to vaccination
- Overtraining syndromes
- Psychiatric conditions including depression
- Drug-induced fatigue, most commonly seen in statins and beta blockers
- Neoplastic disorders including leukaemia, myeloma and lymphoma
- Autoimmune disorders including polymyalgia rheumatica and inflammatory joint disease
- Systemic disease including thyroid disorders, anaemia, diabetes, systemic infections and cardiac disorders.

Investigations for these can be numerous but may include full blood count with differential white cell count, ESR, C-reactive protein, urea and electrolytes including calcium and phosphate, thyroid function and creatine kinase as well as immunoglobulins and electrophoresis.

EXERCISE AND TIREDNESS

'Fatigue', 'tiredness', 'low energy', 'lacking performance' and 'tired all the time' are often complaints or symptoms that athletes present with. To some physicians this may be a heart-sink situation but to others it can be a diagnostic challenge and very satisfying to treat. The differential diagnosis of these types of symptoms is large and detailed analysis is beyond the scope of this book. The list of causes that follows is not exclusive and within this list there are no rarities, as it is possible to have any of these potential diagnoses or, indeed, a combination of them. In simple terms the differential diagnoses can be divided into four sections:

1. Most common causes
   - Overtraining
   - Viral illnesses
   - Dietary causes including, anaemia, vitamin deficiencies and eating disorders, and chronic fatigue syndrome.
2. Less common causes
   - Psychological causes, including anxiety disorders, depression; and sleep abnormalities, including jet lag and drug-induced fatigue (beta blockers, anxiolytics, antidepressants, recreational drugs).
3. Systemic causes
   - Neoplasia including, leukaemias, lymphomas
   - Thyroid disorders
   - Cardiac disorders
   - Anaemia
   - Diabetes
   - Systemic inflammatory disorders, such as colitis or spondyloarthropathies

- Malabsorption disorders including coeliac disease
- Systemic infections including tropical diseases.
4. Others
    - Dehydration
    - Neurological disorders (myasthenia gravis) or stiffness to suggest inflammatory causes.

Details of the patient's drug history, dietary intake and, most importantly, mood, need to be explored. Equally vital is a history of how this patient has been managed in the past, their expectations and the diagnoses they have been given do play a role, not only in assisting diagnosis but maintaining patient compliance.

Examination

On examination there may be very little to find but, despite this, a thorough systemic examination needs to be performed. Although uncommon, stigmata of some systemic disease, such as nail changes in a malabsorption syndrome or a thyroid goitre may previously have been missed. Equally important, it is vital to show the athlete that you are taking their symptoms seriously and that you are leaving no stone unturned in examining them thoroughly. Resting pulse rate is also of importance when compared with normal heart rate and training rate, as is body weight or body fat changes that may be relevant. It is important also not to miss any single or multiple lymph node enlargement, as this may be the only physical sign of some systemic or neoplastic disorder.

Investigations

Obviously, following history and examination, there may be strong pointers as to what the cause may be but, equally there may be no inkling of any possible diagnosis. Often in these cases, a barrage of investigations is performed; however, it is probably acceptable for the following to be performed to cast a wide net.

Full blood picture, ESR, C-reactive protein, infectious mononucleosis test; folic acid and vitamin B levels. Viral studies including coxsackie. U + Es, LTFs, thyroid function, calcium and phosphate; fasting blood sugar and cortisol; iron levels, ferritin, TIBC and transferrin receptor level (normal ferritin greater than 30 ng/mL in females and greater than 50 ng/mL in males, with a transferrin receptor level less than 2.4 mg/L is regarded as normal); coeliac screen, creatine kinase, chest X-ray and spirometry.

Analysis

Hopefully from the above, a diagnosis and plan of action can be formulated. However, there are several conditions that perhaps need further explanation.

Overtraining

This is a common cause of fatigue in athletes, many of whom can spiral down in a desperate effort to improve their symptoms by training more. The symptoms are usually ones of tiredness and worsening performance despite increasing efforts to train, associated with secondary changes of mood disturbance, sleep disturbance and often, frequent viral illnesses. The term 'overreaching' is used by all athletes to describe a transient period when, in response to increased training load, they feel fatigued. However, if accompanied with a rest period it allows an adaptive compensation to build up more persistence and performance with training. If, however, this excess stress is not accompanied by a compensatory and recovery period then overtraining can result, when there is inadequate time to adapt or regenerate to the training load. As mentioned above, if the athlete then continues to train harder and harder, a vicious spiral results, where the athlete's performance deteriorates as they put more effort in. Symptoms of overtraining include fatigue, reduced performance, raised resting heart rate or blood pressure, decreased morning cortisol and a change in the ratio of testosterone to cortisol levels, muscle fatigue, apathy, lack of motivation, sleep disturbance and depression. Although blood tests may suggest this, the most important investigation is looking at the patient's training diary and their periods of rest, which will often give the game away. Management of this problem involves a significant period of rest and down time to assist in recovery and a period of 2 weeks complete rest, followed by weaning into some cross-training can improve symptoms. In addition, a good diet to allow restoration of carbohydrate levels within the muscle and an explanation to the patient and their coach of the condition and its management, usually results in progress. It is important, however, to monitor progress and not to slip back into bad habits, and the patient can assess this themselves with their own monitoring of rest, training and symptom scoring.

Viral illnesses

As has been mentioned before, training with systemic viral illnesses, such as glandular fever, can have deleterious effects. However, what is advised to athletes who have mild viral illnesses, such as upper respiratory tract infections or colds? As a general rule of thumb, physicians should use the 'below the neck' rule. This means that any symptoms from below the level of the neck should perhaps act as a contraindication for intense activity. The explanation for this is that patients with any symptoms confined to above the neck, such as viral sore throat, runny nose, earache, mild headache symptoms, which usually imply mild viral illnesses, should be advised that light training is allowed, as long as the pulse rate is kept below 70% of maximum. For any symptoms below the neck, including elevated temperature, muscle soreness, flu-like symptoms, chest or abdominal symptoms, exercise should be contraindicated for 24 or 48 h until these symptoms have resolved. The evidence for this is that intense exercise with systemic illness may predispose to a worsening of the underlying condition, or the development of myocarditis or chronic fatigue syndrome.

Dietary causes

For more detail on this the reader is referred to the chapter on nutrition. However, it is important to go through a detailed dietary history with the patient to exclude any selective eating, which may include lack of vital ingredients within the diet but also may include a lack of simple and complex carbohydrates. Likewise, causes of folic acid and vitamin D deficiencies and anaemia need to be excluded, some of which may not be dietary but genetic. Finally it is important to exclude an eating disorder, which may be part of the female triad seen in endurance athletes, together with dysfunction of their menstrual periods and osteoporotic risk.

Chronic fatigue syndrome

Chronic fatigue syndrome or myalgic encephalomyelitis (ME) is often defined as a diagnosis of exclusion, having excluded all the possible diagnoses listed above. Unfortunately, there is no one diagnostic test to confirm this condition, which presents as persistent fatigue of more than 6 months duration, associated with four or more of the following: sore throat, lymphadenopathy, myalgia, polyarthropathy, headaches, unsatisfying sleep pattern and post-exercise malaise of more than 24 h, in addition to psychological symptoms including mood changes, memory and concentration disturbance. The cause is unknown and there are several psychological, social and immunological models for the cause. Management of the condition is challenging and can be looked on with despair or with encouragement. My personal approach is to make sure that you take the patient seriously and let them know that. Second is to confirm that they have the diagnosis by excluding any other possible causes as listed above, and to reiterate to the patient that they have this condition and that there is a management plan. This includes correcting any underlying abnormality, be it dietary or psychological, and often the use of antidepressants is helpful in trying to break a cycle of despondency. The mainstay of treatment involves massive patient support and a graduated exercise programme. It is important to inform the patient that they will not wake up one day feeling well if they do nothing now, and that they need to retrain their body totally involving cardiac function, respiratory function, muscle function, hormonal and energy transfer systems to get good results. My advice is to advise them to break the daily functions down into manageable bits, rather than try to complete certain tasks. So, for example, rather than let them exhaust themselves by trying to mow the lawn, they should work out what they can do in terms of mowing the lawn before they feel tired. If this means that they can spread the mowing of the lawn into three separate sessions over 6 days, then this is what they should do, rather than trying to complete the task, exhausting themselves in the process and setting themselves back. Tasks for the day are therefore time-governed rather than task-governed. In this way the patient achieves things, rather than continually fails; and then, progressively increase the time they exercise or perform a function while they improve before fatiguing. This can be done in association with resting heart rate, which is more useful when one returns to actual exercise regimes. The help of the athlete's family, coach and a psychologist and, occasionally, a psychiatrist is essential to a successful recovery.

Take home points

- Always be alert to the presenting symptoms being just one factor in a more generalised systemic illness.
- Be aware of the broad range of possible causes of 'fatigue'.

CLINICAL CASE

A 29-year-old female hockey player presents to your clinic with ongoing right-sided low back pain. This has been present for 6 years, on and off, and initially seemed to have been precipitated when she fell while skiing. She was not severely injured at that time but remembers that as possibly being the cause of her pain. The pain has always been focused around her L4/5 region and radiating into her right buttock, and occasionally, into her upper proximal posterior thigh. Over the last 3 months, her pain has become more severe, radiating into the top of both buttocks, interfering with her daily activity, such as when she sits at work in a call centre. She has seen osteopaths and chiropractors, and a physiotherapist, who have given her a variety of diagnoses and she had an MRI in the past, 5 years ago, when she was seen by an orthopaedic surgeon. The MRI was reported as normal. There are no neurological symptoms in her limbs and no particular night pain, although occasionally her sleep is disturbed. She feels very sore in the morning but finds it easier to get going by doing some stretching exercises in bed and then, in the morning once up, warm her back up. There are no cauda equina symptoms or true radicular symptoms and she is otherwise well, although she had a past history of Achilles tendinopathy in her early 20s. She has no other problems with any other joints and no past history of iritis, bowel disorders or sexually transmitted diseases. There is no relevant past history as far as she is aware; however, her father is awaiting a knee replacement.

- What is the differential diagnosis of the cause of this woman's pain?
- Are there any features in the examination you are going to particularly focus on?

On examination, she is seen to stand with a mildly pronated posture and is slightly overweight. She had reasonable gluteal control on one-legged squat and had no obvious wasting. There was no leg length discrepancy and examination of her back revealed a good degree of flexion but this mainly came from hip flexion and she has hypomobility of her L3/4/5 vertebrae. Extension was particularly limited, reproducing her pain, and showing pivoting at L2, both on extension and lateral flexion. Quadrant or stork test was negative. Examination of her sacroiliac joints showed instability and atypical movement of her right sacroiliac joint. There was no neurological deficit in her lower limbs and her neural tension signs, such as slump and straight leg raise, were normal. Her hip joints were also normal. There was no other joint abnormality, peripherally, but she did have some nail changes in her hands and a small patch of psoriasis over her sacrum and around her umbilicus. Further questioning confirmed that her father's knee replacement was a result of psoriatic monoarthritis that affected him in his 30s, resulting in an osteoarthritic knee. Palpation of her back revealed hypomobility and tenderness over her L4/5 vertebrae, and there was discomfort over her right sacroiliac joint and on pelvic squeeze test. There was no abnormality in her facet joints for iliolumbar ligaments.

- What is the most likely diagnosis and how would you investigate this patient?

It seems possible that this patient is presenting with the early signs of sacroiliitis and may have some inflammatory bone disease or early spondyloarthropathy. Investigations should include lumbar spine and pelvis X-ray, and inflammatory blood tests including full blood picture, ESR and C-reactive protein. As has been discussed elsewhere in this book, screening test with HLA, B27 and autoimmune profile at this stage may not be appropriate. While the investigations are underway, it would be appropriate to give her a trial of antiinflammatory medication, to see if this could benefit her symptoms. The results come back showing normal X-rays, particularly, with no signs of sacroiliitis, but also no signs of facet joint dysfunction; however, her blood tests confirm a raised ESR and C-reactive protein, but normal full blood count. She returns showing significant improvement with her antiinflammatories, and asks about her subsequent treatment.

- Are there any other investigations you would now perform and how would you best manage this patient?

At this stage it may be difficult to be prescriptive about her management. It may well be that she has a mild inflammatory sacroiliitis that can be managed with antiinflammatories, episodically, and good physiotherapy, maintaining her range of movement, and core stability strength. However, her symptoms need to be monitored carefully, mainly, in the form of assessing the severity of early morning symptoms and range of movement; further assessment with an MRI scan may confirm the information within her right sacroiliac joint, and the physiotherapist also needs to monitor her range of movement, to be alert to the onset of any developing spondylolytic picture. Localised pain can be managed with a CT-guided corticosteroid injection into the sacroiliac joint; however, it would be very useful to incorporate the help of a rheumatologist early on in this patient's condition, to prevent any progression, and to be alert to any peripheral joint disease.

REFERENCES

1. Anderson SD. Exercise induced asthma. In: Middleton E Jr, Reed CE, Ellis EF, et al., eds. Allergy: Principles and practice. 4th edn. St Louis MO: Mosby; 1993:1343–1367.

2. Godfrey S. Exercise-induced asthma. In: Barnes PJ, Grunstein MM, Leff AR, Woolcock AJ, eds. Asthma. Philadelphia PA: Lippincott-Raven; 1997:1105–1120.

3. Rupp NT. Diagnosis and management of exercise-induced asthma. Phys Sportsmed 1996; 24(1):77–87.

4. Martin JB, Ruskin J. Faintness, syncope and seizures. In: Isselbacher KJ, Braunwald E, Wilson JD, eds. Harrison's principles of internal medicine. 13th edn. Columbus OH: McGraw-Hill Inc; 1994:134–140.

5. Garson A, Jr. Arrhythmias and sudden cardiac death in elite athletes. American College of Cardiology, 16th Bethesda Conference. Pediatr Med Chir 1998; 20(2):101–103.

6. Maron BJ. Hypertrophic cardiomyopathy. Practical steps for preventing sudden death. Phys Sportsmed 2002; 30(1):19–24

7. Epstein SE, Maron BJ. Sudden death and the competitive athlete: perspectives on preparticipation screening studies. J Am Coll Cardiol 1986; 7(1):220–230.

8. Glorioso J Jr, Reeves M. Marfan syndrome; screening for sudden death in athletes. Curr Sports Med Rep 2002; 1(2):67–74.

9. Shawdon A. Gastro-oesophageal reflux and exercise. Important pathology to consider in the athletic population. Sports Med 1995; 20(2):109–116.

10. Rao SS, Beaty J, Chamberlain M et al. Effects of acute graded exercise on human colonic motility. Am J Physiol 1999; 276(5 Part 1):G1221–G1226.

11. Moy CS, Songer TJ, LaPorte RE, et al. IDDM: physical activity and death. Am J Epidemiol 1993; 137(1):74–81.

12. Colberg SR, Swain DP. Exercise and diabetes control: A winning combination. Phys Sportsmed 2000; 28(4):63–81.

13. McCrory PR, Berkovic SF. Concussive convulsions. Incidence in sport and treatment recommendations. Sports Med 1998; 25(2):131–136.

14. Kim TH, Uhm WS, Inman RD. Pathogenesis of ankylosing spondylitis and reactive arthritis. Curr Opin Rheumatol 2005; 17(4):400–405.

Index